Natural Treatment of Allergies

Natural Treatment of
Allergies

Learn How to Treat
Your Allergies with Safe, Natural Methods

Dr. Ramon Roselló

with

Anna Huete

Translated by **Allie Hauptman**

Skyhorse Publishing

Skyhorse Publishing books may be purchased in bulk at special discounts for sales promotion, corporate gifts, fund-raising, or educational purposes. Special editions can also be created to specifications. For details, contact the Special Sales Department, Skyhorse Publishing, 307 West 36th Street, 11th Floor, New York, NY 10018 or info@skyhorsepublishing.com.

Skyhorse® and Skyhorse Publishing® are registered trademarks of Skyhorse Publishing, Inc.®, a Delaware corporation.

Visit our website at www.skyhorsepublishing.com.

10 9 8 7 6 5 4 3 2 1

Library of Congress Cataloging-in-Publication Data is available on file.

Cover design by Qualcom Design
Cover photo credit Thinkstock

ISBN: 978-1-62914-467-2

E-book ISBN: 978-1-63220-059-4

Printed in the United States of America

Contents

Introduction

"Health is within you, and you don't see it;
illness is within you, and you don't realize."

— SUFI PROVERB

These days, allergies complicate the daily life of many people, children and adults alike, and present a challenge for health professionals.

One day, a harmless substance that you regularly encounter in the air, in what you touch, or what you eat, becomes your worst enemy. From this moment on, any future contact with this substance will provoke an allergic reaction, forcing you to change your daily habits in many ways.

Pollen, dust mites, animal dander, mold, foods, certain metals, medicines...All of these things are found in almost every house, and on the street in every town and city. And any one, or ones, of these can be the cause of your asthma, your hay fever, your topical dermatitis, or your food intolerance. You have become an allergic person, and this reality will seem like a life sentence.

This is the feeling that many people who suffer from allergies have, because no one can give them a scientific explanation of this disorder that came out of nowhere, without warning.

Conventional medicine can explain what happens when someone develops an allergy: an error is made by your immune system. But they don't know why it happens.

There seems to be a hereditary component, it seems that the disease itself chooses where to settle, it seems that children grow out of their allergies, but it also seems that they are difficult to cure in adulthood…

One indisputable fact is that allergies are spreading without control, and more people suffer from allergies all the time. Facts show that modern life aids considerably in this, together with, for example, pollution, cigarette smoke, stress, bad health, a sedentary lifestyle, and a lack of exposure to nature. It is not to be overlooked that there is a much greater presence of allergies in urban environments but not so much in rural areas, despite the higher concentrations of pollen, animal dander, mold, and dust mites.

Meanwhile, those who suffer from allergies search for relief and, above all, results. Sometimes this is done using conventional medicine, and other times, more and more often, through natural remedies. The best thing is to know how to take advantage of the benefits of all of these methods and combine conventional and alternative medicines into one single treatment that restores your health through various approaches.

Conventional medicine offers you relief from annoying symptoms with the use of drugs and allergy vaccines. The side effects are inevitable, but the relief is undeniable. And, above all, you should never refuse conventional medicine in serious cases like anaphylactic shock or a bad asthma attack, because it can save your life.

On the other hand, natural therapies offer you the possibility of thoroughly healing yourself. It may seem like an exaggeration, but thousands of years of experience speak to their effectiveness. Naturopathy, homeopathy, acupuncture, Bach flower remedies, yoga, and meditation are some of the ways to reestablish the balance between your body and mind. All of these forms of therapy achieve positive, and even spectacular results when it comes to the treatments of allergies, and you don't have to limit yourself to just one. On the contrary, it has been shown that when you combine them, their synergy augments the benefits and your body recovers much more rapidly.

Nor can we neglect to say that they are not just therapies, but they can provide the backdrop for a new lifestyle where your first priority is your physical and emotional well-being. Sometimes illness becomes the direct route to reconnecting with yourself and emphasizes the importance of the things you have. Through the search for a cure, many people have found themselves, and have found a new meaning in their life.

On this long journey to overcoming illness, we will try to provide you with a roadmap to explain what is happening to you, how it is happening, and what you can do to fix it. This is the goal of the following pages, and we hope that they help you understand what allergies are, what it means to live with them, and how to confront the symptoms and their origins.

What Are Allergies?

Allergies can be defined differently depending on if we look at them through the fields of academic medicine, natural medicine, or traditional Chinese medicine. What we have no doubt about is that it is a growing phenomenon that can create a lot of discomfort and show us that our sophisticated immune system can have inexplicable faults that cause excessive reactions to inoffensive stimuli. According to many experts, the existence of allergies is the price societies in developing countries have to pay, since it is in those places that there are a prolific number of cases.

In effect, what is troublesome is that allergies continue to affect more and more people. The number of people with allergies grows, most of all in industrialized countries. Moreover, there are many people who are not even aware that they are suffering from any ailment. The symptoms multiply and are no longer limited to rhinitis or hay fever, asthma, and eczema, but they can also include fatigue, migraines, depression, dizziness, discomfort, arrhythmias, weight-loss, constipation, diarrhea, rheumatism, and hyperactivity in children.

The most common manifestations of allergies are asthma, rhinitis or hay fever, dermatitis, and food allergies. As their origins are not always clear, treatment through conventional medicine is a very complicated process and is reduced to an attempt to relieve the symptoms produced by the allergic reaction. Because of this, the number of people affected by allergies who seek natural remedies continues to grow; these are remedies that treat the person rather than focusing on the illness. Alternative therapies intend to regain the balance within our bodies and help restore the immune system's correct function. In many cases, the results are surprising.

Defining Allergies

Allergies are excessive reactions within our body. That's it, in short, but there are many factors that are still inexplicable in many cases.

Basically, our body reacts inappropriately to external substances that are harmless to the majority of people. These allergenic substances, called "allergens," can be found both in nature and in chemicals and generate a disproportionate response in our immune system. They reach our bodies through inhalation, ingestion, or skin contact.

Our immune system is responsible for allergic reactions. It is made up of a collection of cells that circulate through the blood and form parts of different organs. Its mission is simple: to recognize foreign elements that enter our body and organize the defense against them. This reaction is called the "immune response." Thanks to this, our immune system recognizes bacteria and viruses, problematic agents in our bodies, as causes of infection. If it weren't for our immune system, any infection, even a cold, could have fatal consequences due to its ability to spread without any resistance.

Nevertheless, although the immune response is very important, it can occasionally cause us serious problems, and even death. These problems include autoimmune diseases where our immune systems confuse components of our bodies for foreign elements and initiate a response against them, like in cases of rheumatism. It also creates complications for people who have had an organ transplant. Their immune defenses identify the newly transplanted organ as foreign and begin to fight it, causing a rejection if medicine is not administered to diminish the reaction.

The final and most common problem that can provoke a false immune reaction is the issue of allergies. In normal circumstances, our immune system is our guardian and is always alert to anything harmful that enters our body. However, in a person who suffers from allergies, the immune system reacts incorrectly to harmless substances that it considers dangerous, and develops a pathological process that is difficult to diagnose and fix.

An Old Ailment with a Recent History

Even though allergies can seem to us to be a modern ailment, the truth is that their story can be traced through many years of history.

In the time of the ancient Egyptians, there was a pharaoh who fell victim to a wasp sting, and in the 5th century B.C., Hippocrates documented the existence of people who were "hostile" to cheese, a food that was not compatible with their bodies. And in this era, at the beginning of the 16th century, the Roman cardinal Olivieri Caraffi prohibited the entrance of anyone carrying flowers because they made him sick.

However, it took four more centuries for doctors to consider allergies to be a common ailment, though their origins remained a mystery. In 1903, pediatricians Clemens von Pirquet and Béla Schick discovered a successful path of research, and postulated that the cause of this illness, which they called an "allergy," resides in the formation of antibodies that instead of defending the organism, attack and harm it.

➤

One year later, Charles Richet and Paul Portier realized that if you administer the venom of a sea anemone to a dog, it won't be affected the first time, but the dog would die upon the third dose. They called this phenomenon "anaphylaxis," or a lack of defenses. Their discovery was a great help to future scientists and won Charles Richet the Nobel Prize in 1913.

In 1996, Swedish scientist Gunner Johansson and the husband and wife team Kimishige and Teruko Ishizaka of Japan discovered that the antibody that provokes allergies is immunoglobulin E (IgE).

Since then, research continues to unravel the mysteries of this strange auto-immune disease, and moves toward revealing its origin as well as its prevention.

A Scientific Explanation We will try to explain in simple scientific terms the biological process that takes place in our body when having an allergy attack.

The principal cells that make up our immune system are macrophages and lymphocytes T and B. When these come in contact with a substance that our body identifies as foreign or as an allergen, they initiate a series of reactions until molecules called "immunoglobulins" (Ig), or antibodies, are formed, that join with the allergen and achieve its destruction and elimination through various mechanisms.

The immune system of the allergic person begins to construct this immunoglobulin from the first exposure to an allergen, but only shows the symptom of an allergy when the productions of these immunoglobulins have exceeded their tolerance limit. That is to say that time can pass between the first exposure to the allergen and the allergic reaction. However, once this tolerance has been exceeded, any new contact with the allergy, no matter how insignificant, will produce the symptoms of the allergy. This is the explanation for how one day a substance that we had been living with or ingesting habitually can suddenly cause an asthma attack or eczema.

These immunoglobulins that our body makes in response to an allergen react only to this concrete allergen. That is to say, they are specific immunoglobulins or IgE. However, different types of a specific immunoglobulin can be produced at a time, which means it is possible to be allergic to more than one substance. And, what's more, it can produce crossed reactions, which means that the same type of IgE reacts to seemingly different substances, like dust mites and seafood. If you have an allergy to dust, it is possible that you're also allergic to seafood, because both contain a protein called "tropomyosin" which is the allergen that produces the allergic reaction. So, even though they are seemingly different substances, they produce the same type of symptoms.

There are five different types of immunoglobulins or antibodies that our bodies produce: IgG, IgA, IgM, IgD, and IgE. However, only IgE is responsible for the reactions that provoke asthma and the majority of allergic reactions.

HUNTING AND TRAPPING

The IgE that our body produces are attached to mastocytes, cells that contain granules of histamine and other allergy mediators that are produced in the nose, eyes, lungs, and gastrointestinal system. IgE adheres to the surface of the mastocytes in order to "trap" its respective allergen. When the allergen enters the body, IgE attracts it and they lock together like a lock and key. The IgE sends a signal to the mastocyte to defend itself against the invader, causing it to release histamine. This hormone, histamine, is what causes redness, swelling, and excessive secretions from the skin and mucous membranes. These symptoms can provoke asthma, diarrhea, rhinitis, or hives, depending on the zone where the body is fighting the allergen.

What Does Histamine Do?

Histamine is a hormone with a basic vasodilatory function, causing inflammation and irritation during an allergic reaction.

However, it has other functions that are important and beneficial to our bodies, provided it is secreted in appropriate amounts for each case.

For example, thanks to its vasodilatory properties, histamine modulates blood pressure and partly controls the heart's electrical activity. It is also present in our digestive system and regulates the secretion of gastric juices. Also, it is an important neurotransmitter in the central nervous system and has many different functions in the brain.

Therefore, it is not localized to a specific organ or zone in our body. However, as with every part of our organism, its job is important and, without a doubt, indispensable to the proper function of our body.

Depending on the type of allergic substance and the form of exposure, the immune system's response can range from being insignificant to being very serious. And even though the majority of allergic reactions are benign, some can become fatal, like anaphylactic shock.

We are all exposed to many potentially allergic substances, and most of us can live with them without presenting any symptoms. That is to say, we don't exceed our tolerance limit because we aren't predisposed to suffer allergies.

On the contrary, for people who have an allergy, the substance will trigger a reaction every time they come in contact with it. What's worse is that it only takes the smallest amount of the allergen for the allergic reaction to take place.

The Allergic Cascade. Normally an allergic reaction takes place immediately upon contact with the allergen, but many cases exist where that is not the case. The mediatory substances that are released during a crisis, like histamine, not only affect the surrounding tissues, but also recruit the leucocytes that contribute to the name "late phase response" that appears after several hours.

An immediate reaction lasts about two hours and is caused by mastocytes. A slow or late phase response is one that appears about six hours after exposure to the allergen and is caused by basophils and eosinophils that release cytokines and chemokines. Because of this, many allergists agree that the allergic individual usually has a two-phase reaction, or, in other words, an allergic cascade.

This second, new release of histamine in the body has not been studied until relatively recently and caused much confusion when it came time to determine the allergens that trigger the reaction. Its most notable effect is that it prolongs inflammation for hours, so that a bout of rhinitis can end up lasting days, even though the exposure to the allergen had been isolated; thus, the mucous membrane remains inflamed, and the symptoms remain. Sometimes this is the difference between chronic and seasonal rhinitis.

The late phase response is especially virulent in people who suffer from asthma. There have been cases in which after receiving urgent medical attention that stabilizes the crisis, the patient suffers a new, stronger reaction right after returning home. The cytokines and chemokines that produce this late response are much stronger than histamines.

During this late phase, the allergic symptoms related to inflammation return chronically and their treatment is even more complicated. What's more, a person can become hyperreactive. If you are allergic to dust mites and you suffer this late phase reaction, it is probable that environmental factors, cigarette smoke, perfumes, or the fumes from fresh paint can cause a new reaction. It's not that you are allergic to these products, but that because your mucous membrane remains inflamed as a result of the eosinophils, a minimally irritating agent can trigger a new attack.

Allergic March. When symptoms of allergies appear, they usually cause rhinitis, eczema, or asthma attacks. These symptoms tell us that our immune system is reacting poorly, and this manifests itself in the form of illness.

Nevertheless, with every further exposure to the allergen, it is more common for the reaction to not be limited to only these ailments. As time passes and the number of exposures to the allergens responsible for our ailments grows, our body is going to yield and begin what is called an "allergic march."

This term defines the situation of people who, for example, begin to suffer from eczema and then after a certain time, begin to show additional symptoms of rhinitis. That is to say, allergies spread through our bodies and are not limited to just one manifestation. Among these most common cases is rhinitis complicated by asthma.

Because of this, it is necessary to try to detect which allergens produce a reaction in your body and to find a remedy, preferably a natural one, to this situation that is a great health risk.

Chronic Illness. As we have seen, the cause of an allergy can't always be attributed to a concrete substance, but rather to the individual. Certain people are genetically predisposed to develop an exaggerated reaction after repeated contact with substances that are harmless to most people, but potentially capable of inducing a defensive reaction in the body.

Increase in Allergies

One in every five people in the US suffers from allergies, or 60 million people. Allergies have been increasing since the 1980s across various demographics.

-Asthma and Allergy Foundation of America

Nowadays, more than 15 percent of the worldwide population is allergic to one substance or another, and in most cases, allergic to more than one at the time. There is no clear explanation for why some people develop this kind of reaction, but it seems to be that genetics play an important role in this development. It is not the allergy itself that is passed on, but rather the predisposition to develop an allergy. If one parent has allergies, their child has a 48 percent chance of having allergies as well. If both parents have allergies, the probability of the offspring developing allergies grows by 70 percent. What's more, allergies can develop at any age, and it is not uncommon for people older than forty years to one day start sneezing, get tested, and discover that they have become an allergic person.

The emotional state of the person also plays an important role in the development of an allergy. Asthma can be caused by stress, depression, or a crisis; rhinitis can be produced by a trauma, and nerves and stress can aggravate atopic dermatitis and food intolerances. It is key to take care of our bodies and emotions to attain complete balance, and natural therapies can aid greatly in this process.

Pseudoallergies and Food Intolerances

These terms refer to allergic problems that are caused by different processes from an allergic reaction. Their effects on the patient, however, are the same as you would find in an allergic person, and can produce asthma, rhinitis, dermatitis, and diarrhea without the intervention of IgE.

In these cases, our bodies produce antibodies IgA and, after multiple stimuli, IgG or immunoglobulin G. The IgG are the same kind that are produced against proteins of microorganisms and that give us the acquired immunity. Their stimulus and constant production is the scientific base for vaccines.

Different from the immediate allergic reaction that takes place within two or three hours of the initial stimulus, when the pseudoallergic process is produced through IgG, the antigen or allergen does not usually produce an immediate and evident reaction, but rather it produces disorders whose origins are difficult to trace and have less specific characteristics. Intolerances that are provoked by a certain food decrease our intestinal flora, causing our intestines to become more permeable and unprotected. With every exposure to the offensive food, the intestine has greater difficulty releasing proteins. This causes the entire protein to pass through the intestine into our body, which consequently creates antibodies, a type of substance that our immune system is not accustomed to manage. This process can take weeks, months, or even years, and will provoke symptoms that are less identifiable, making it difficult to discover the origin of our illness.

This causes specific foods, food additives, or medicines to produce certain IgG as a defense against some of these characteristic proteins, and new antigens. That is to say, every time we eat this food or foods again, the IgG is produced. In some cases, there are digestive problems or diarrhea, but often, these symptoms of moderate or chronic ailments are more discrete and hard to trace back to the specific food. These can be dermatologic problems like psoriasis, pruritus, eczema, or acne; respiratory problems like asthma or rhinitis that usually overlap with allergic reactions produced by IgE; neurological problems like headaches, vertigo, migraines, or dizziness; psychological ailments like fatigue, nausea, anxiety, depression, or child hyperactivity; gastrointestinal issues like constipation, diarrhea, irritable bowel syndrome, abdominal swelling, or pain; and including complications with other illnesses like arthritis, fibromyalgia, or chronic fatigue syndrome.

As you can see, it is not treated like an allergy but the consequences are identical and its causes are difficult to determine. There are some tests to check for food intolerances that will be explained later in the chapter about allergy tests.

Differences Between an Allergic Reaction and a Pseudoallergy:

IgE	IgG
Immediate showing of symptoms	Slower onset symptoms
Type I reactions	Repress II, III, and IV reactions
Positive to cutaneous tests	Negative to tests
Few foods involved	Many foods involved
Small traces of a substance can trigger a reaction	It takes larger amounts to trigger a reaction
Reactions mainly in skin and mucous membranes	Reactions in all tissues
More common in children	More common in adults
Sometimes sensed by the patient	Not sensed by the patient
Recommended diet eliminating the offending food	More difficult to reconfigure the diet
Exclusion of the substance will solve the problem	Exclusion will improve the problem
Almost never able to return to tolerating the substance.	Sometimes over time you're able to tolerate the food again.

Food Intolerances Not Linked to IgE/IgG. To further complicate the situation, there are also many food intolerances that do not correspond to any process involving the allergic mechanisms mediated by IgE or IgG. These pseudoallergies act directly against the mastocytes, triggering the release of histamine in its direct form, without the mediation of the specific allergy antibodies. This reaction is usually provoked by a number of medicines, especially acetylsalicylic acid, which is commonly found in our home first aid kits.

Pseudoallergies are also triggered by chemical additives or impurities in foods, like colorings, preservatives, flavor enhancers, pesticide residues, sulfites in dried fruits, anti-mildew agents, and prepared potato products; or in foods rich in histamines like cheese and wines, among others.

These elements only trigger an allergic reaction in people who are especially sensitive and go undetected in the usual allergy tests and in the analytics that search for the antibodies IgE. Nevertheless, as in the case of a pseudoallergy, it is helpful to test problems with digestion.

Regardless of the reaction to the trigger, the consequences for the patient are the same, so we will treat them the same way.

Among the most important cases, we cite:

- Intolerance of milk due to a deficit of intestinal lactase.
- Intolerances due to vasoactive amines (tyramine and histamine) present in certain foods: fermented cheese, alcohol, tuna, sausages, smoked sausages, fermented cabbage.
- Intolerances to food additives: sulfites contained in certain wines (headaches) or glutamate (commonly used in Chinese cuisine).
- Intolerances due to pesticides, preservatives, food colorings, and additives in general.

What are the symptoms of allergies?

Even though an allergic reaction can manifest itself in many ways, the problems caused by histamine come from three specific actions: inflammation, vasodilation, and redness.

However, the symptoms that trigger these three reactions are varied as a function of the structure on which histamine is released.

Below are the principal allergic symptoms and the type of allergy that can produce them. However, this is only an indication, and if you have a cough it does not necessarily mean you are having an asthma attack. If, on the contrary, you suffer from more than one of these symptoms, it is possible that you are suffering from one of the types of allergies that we discussed.

Symptom	Type of Allergy
Cough	Asthma, hay fever or rhinitis, food allergy, allergy to medicine
Sneeze	Hay fever or rhinitis
Difficulty Breathing	Asthma, food allergy, allergy to medicine
Sibilant breathing	Asthma
Nasal congestion	Hay fever or rhinitis
Acute secretion of mucous	Hay fever or rhinitis
Itching in eyes, throat and mouth	Hay fever or rhinitis, food allergy
Skin irritation, itching, and swelling	Allergy to medicine, allergy to insect bite, allergy to chemical products
Stomach ache	Food allergy
Indigestion	Food allergy
Feeling of burning in the stomach	Food allergy
Redness, pain, or swelling of the joints	Food allergy, allergy to medicine, allergy to chemical products

Symptom	Type of Allergy
Headache	Hay fever or rhinitis, allergy to chemical products
Fatigue	Hay fever or rhinitis, asthma, allergy to chemical products

Types of Allergic Reactions

Allergists classify allergic reactions in four different types. Each one of these has its own characteristics and symptoms.

- **Type I:** Acute reactions with immediate hypersensitivity, mediated by antibodies IgE.
- **Type II:** Induces cellular destruction. Presence of antibodies IgG. Slow fixation on the cellular surface like, for example, the intestinal villi.
- **Type III:** Presence of immunocomplexes Ag-Ac (IgG in the blood circulation that can be deposited in the intestinal mucous and other tissues).
- **Type IV:** Delayed hypersensitivity. Presence of T lymphocytes with chronic inflammation (IgG).

In a Type I reaction, IgE are responsible for the reaction. Alternately, in the remaining three types, the symptoms are provoked by IgG, responsible for pseudoallergies as we described before.

Among the generalized Type I allergies are the following:

- **Immediate difficulty breathing.**
- **Possibility of anaphylactic shock.** This is the most serious allergic reaction. In this reaction, the blood vessels dilate and

become permeable to liquid, so that much of what they contain is transferred to the tissues. This causes blood pressure to drop, which can result in circulatory collapse, apnea, and death.

Localized reactions can be produced.

- **Skin:** hives, Quincke's edema, atopic dermatitis.
- **Respiratory mucous:** asthma, cough, rhinitis.
- **Digestive mucous:** acqueous diarrhea.
- **Mucous in mouth and throat.**

Allergic reactions II, III, and IV are mediated by IgG and their symptoms are usually the following:

- **Digestive:** heartburn, mouth ulcers, gastritis, colitis, constipation, diarrhea, nausea.
- **Respiratory:** cough, bronchitis, asthma.
- **Joints:** joint pain, joint stiffness.
- **General:** migraines, fatigue, depression, obesity.

Not all hypersensitive reactions fit this model. In fact, there are actually many skin allergies provoked by medicines that are an enigma for specialists, as is the case with Lyell's syndrome. Moreover, there are many medicines that provoke pseudoallergies, that is to say, that their active ingredients occasionally cause allergic reactions without the immune system producing specific immunoglobulins.

What are allergens?

We have explained that the immune system is the defense mechanism of our bodies and that it protects us from innumerable substances that are present in the air we breathe, in what we eat, and in what we touch. The term allergen refers to any element among this huge group. The only requirement for a substance to qualify as an allergen is that it triggers an allergic response in an individual. The substance that the allergic body considers foreign is harmless on its own, but it is characterized by having a determined size. The substances usually are made up of proteins.

They can also be substances that are present in food additives or medicines. Even though their molecules consist of relatively few atoms, these bind with a protein produced by our body, making them large enough to cause a false alarm.

Throughout the documented history of allergies, there has been shown to be a consistent group of common allergies. Among them are pollen, dust mites in the home, mold, certain medicines, insect venom, and other animal substances, like saliva and urine. With respect to food, those that produce the most allergies are milk, eggs, fish, shellfish, dried fruit, stone fruit, and chocolate.

All of these allergies can be identified through certain allergy tests, but there are many which escape this analysis, as they are traced back to fumes emitted by factories or detergents.

Allergies can also be classified by their way of entering our body. If they are inhaled allergens they produce respiratory allergies like asthma and hay fever. This group includes plant pollen, dust mites, and mold. Contact allergens produce dermatitis or eczema. They are substances that trigger a local allergic reaction only by touching the skin. Among these are detergents, cosmetics, hard water, metals, and certain plants.

Lastly are allergens that include ingested foods and medicines. Pharmaceuticals that often trigger allergic reactions include certain antibiotics, especially aspirin and penicillin, which is a fungus. Vitamins and local anesthetics can also trigger an allergic reaction. In fact, whatever medicine is a potential allergen depends on the metabolism of each person. This possibility grows enormously if one abuses its consumption. This can result in severe anaphylactic shock, that is to say, as generalized inflammation that causes respiratory problems, loss of consciousness, and even death. The reason is that many of these substances are administered intravenously or intramuscularly, making the intensity of the immune response much more pronounced. Anaphylactic shock is infrequent and affects many organs at once. It begins with itching on the feet and hands, general rash, difficulty breathing, and cardiocirculatory collapse. It requires immediate medical attention. Anaphylaxis can also be produced by contact allergens, like insect bites, or certain foods.

Diagnosing
Allergies

The first step to successfully treating an allergy is to understand its origin and what allergen is provoking this reaction in our body.

This first fundamental step allows us to obtain a diagnosis and a treatment. A specialist must understand the patient's background and their environment and workplace. They perform a thorough physical examination and ask questions about possible hereditary factors, specific symptoms in certain moments, daily life, diet, pets, workplace, and many more.

However, besides the personal environmental factors of the patient, there are other diagnostic tools that can help us understand the origin of the symptoms.

There are two types of diagnostic approaches. One involves performing blood tests that we will describe in this chapter, and the other approach relies on skin tests. These tests determine the presence of antibodies in the patient and also identify which allergens are triggering the allergic reaction.

Blood Tests

There are three blood tests that are regularly performed. Two tests determine the presence of antibodies, either in the blood or in the blood serum.

The third is used to analyze a very broad spectrum of foods, and allows for a greater exploration than is examined in skin tests. The food intolerance test helps find the origin of certain food allergens that until now have passed unnoticed and are the basis for the majority of undiagnosed allergies.

RAST Test. When a person suspects they have developed an allergy, the first test administered is a radioallergosorbent test. This complicated-sounding test is no more than a blood analysis to determine the concentration of immunoglobulins E and G.

This test consists of combining small samples of the patient's blood in test tubes with different allergens. In the case of an actual allergy, the blood produces antibodies to combat the foreign protein. The test only serves as an indication that an allergy exists, and does not determine the degree of sensitivity to the allergen causing the reaction. But if IgE or other immunoglobulins are discharged, this is sufficient motive to certify that the patient's symptoms are caused by an allergy. In certain cases they can even double from what is normally produced.

In the case that the analysis yields a positive result, other diagnostic tests will be performed whose objective is to try and understand what type of substance or allergen is provoking the allergic reaction.

Test to determine the CLA allergen-specific IgE. In this test, the patient's blood serum is analyzed. The objective is the same as the RAST test, but the constant, in this case, is the serum instead of the blood.

The samples are put in contact with specific allergens to check the levels of immunoglobulins through an in vitro process in the lab.

Food Intolerance Test. This test consists of an analysis of the patient's blood. Once the sample is obtained, it is tested in a lab where they re-create the reaction between the blood cells and 100 of the most common foods in our diet, as well as 20 of the most commonly used colorings and preservatives found in the supermarket.

■ **Foods:** almonds, apples, apricots, artichokes, asparagus, avocado, baker's yeast, bananas, barley, beetroot sugar, black pepper, brewer's yeast, broccoli, butter, cabbage, cane sugar, carrots, cauliflower, celery, cheese, cherries, chicken, chickpeas, chilies, cinnamon, clams, cocoa, coconut, cod, coffee, corn, cow's milk, crab, cucumber, duck, egg white, egg yolk, eggplant, flounder, garlic, goat's milk, grapefruit, grapes, green beans, hake, halibut, hazelnut, honey, kiwis, kola nut, lamb, leek, lemon, lentils, lettuce, lobster, malt, melon, millet, mushroom, mussels, mustard, oats, olives, onion, orange, oyster, parsley, peach, peanut, pear, peas, peppers, pineapples, pinto beans, plums, pork, potato, rabbit, rape, rice, rye, salmon, sardines, sesame, shrimp, soy, spinach, strawberries, sunflowers, tea, tomatoes, trout, tuna, veal, walnut, watermelon, wheat, yam, zucchini.

■ **Additives and Colorings:** aspartame (E951), benzoic acid (E210), monosodium glutamate (MSG) (E621) polysorbate 80 (E422), potassium nitrate (E252), potassium nitride (E249), saccharine (E954), sorbic acid (E200), sodium metabisulfite (E223), sodium sulfate (E221), tartrazine (E102), quinoline yellow (E104), brilliant scarlet (E124), amaranth (E123), erythrosine (E127), patent blue (E131), indigo carmine (E132), green 5 (E142), sunset yellow FCF (E110), brilliant black (E151).

In this test, the behavior of the patient's immune system is analyzed when the sample is exposed in vitro to each of these foods and chemicals. The reactivity to any of these gives guidelines to determine which ones act as an allergen in our bodies.

The test can give a "high positive," "medium positive," or "low positive." In the first case, the patient must eliminate the identified food from their diet for a minimum of two years, in the second case, for six months, and in the third, for a couple of weeks. Then the patient can begin to reintroduce the food into their diet in controlled amounts, observing the possible symptoms or their absence.

With the information that this test provides about our metabolism with respect to possible intolerances or food sensitivities, a nutritionist can personalize our diet and notably improve our quality of life.

As we have mentioned previously, this is not about the allergy, but rather the substances that are absorbed by our intestine and that allow whole proteins to pass into our bodies, which provoke a pseudoallergic reaction and show symptoms identical to an allergy.

A nutritional specialist can approach problems like gastrointestinal disorders, rhinitis, asthma, certain types of dermatitis, chronic fatigue, obesity, water retention, headaches, arthritis, constipation, bloating, etc., from a dietary point of view. Foods and chemical products present in common diets are analyzed in tests for dietary intolerances conducted in laboratories.

Skin Tests

In these types of tests, the goal is to reproduce on the skin the kind of reaction that takes place in the organs where the symptoms of the allergy occur, like the epidermis or lungs. This is possible because the skin contains the same type of special cells, or masto-cytes, that are located in the nostrils, digestive and respiratory systems, and in the case of an allergic person, also contain IgE antibodies that react against the present allergens and mediate the release of histamine.

Even though the reliability of skin tests is not absolute, they allow the patient to get a diagnosis in many cases of respiratory and topical allergies, penicillin, insect bites, and foods. They are very adequate in the case of a pollen allergy, but less reliable when the allergens are foods, animal dander, mold, or dust mites.

It is always necessary to see a professional specialist, as there is a risk of anaphylactic shock if the quantity of allergens is too great, or the results could give false positives or negatives if the adequate amount is not administered.

Skin prick or scratch test. The scratch test is one of the most common testing methods.

It consists of putting a small amount of the suspected aller-gen on the skin of the forearm, bicep, or spine. Next, the skin is scratched to allow the substance to be introduced into the body. The skin is carefully observed for signs of a reaction, specifically swelling or redness of the affected area, or an outbreak of hives, called a "flare reaction."

The results are generally obtained within about twenty min-utes and many suspected allergens can be tested for at the same time.

If hives have developed, they will last about a half hour before disappearing, as the quantity of the introduced allergen is very small.

Prick Test Technique for Allergy Tests. In this test, a drop of the allergen is deposited on the skin, and a small puncture is made on top of it with a needle. The test is usually administered on the skin of the inner forearm and multiple allergens are tested at once. The skin is marked with a pen or felt-tipped marker to identify the site of each test and allergen.

To avoid a false result, two other small punctures are made with histamine and saline. Unreactive skin will show a slight reaction to the histamine, the same as if the patient is treated with antihistamines, which they should stop taking at least a week before taking the test. Therefore the results would be unrepresentative. If the saline provokes a visible reaction, the patient has particularly sensitive skin. In both cases, the results of the tests would little serve the specialist.

When the small amount of the allergen has penetrated the skin, it will trigger a reaction in the sensitized cells and release histamine that will cause the formation of hives surrounded by an itchy reddish area.

After 15 minutes, the results will appear and the hives can be measured. It is a painless and safe test.

Intradermal Test. This is also a test done on the forearm, but in this case, a small dose of the allergen is injected below the surface of the skin with a fine needle. This method administers a greater quantity of the allergen than the other tests and is used to determine the reaction to a certain allergen.

It is usually used when the previous tests yield a negative result.

Patch Test. This test is used to identify the allergens responsible for allergic dermatitis. Small patches injected with a small amount of the suspected allergen or allergens are applied to the back. They are placed in rows all across the back and covered with an adhesive bandage. The patches are kept on the back for 48 hours and the patient needs to follow a set of precautions to avoid altering the results; keep the area dry, avoid heat and sweat, do not scratch the area, and do not expose it to light.

After 48 hours, the skin is marked with a felt-tipped pen, the patches are removed, and the first stage is complete. After another 72 to 96 hours, the second stage is also completed.

The test is administered in groups of allergens and as a rule begins with a panel of 29 allergens that correspond to the European standard. On another side, allergens that usually cause contact allergies are introduced. Also, if a founded suspicion exists, there are specific panels for different professions and substances they come in contact with often (cosmetics, metals, etc).

Mucosal Test. In this case, the allergen is applied to the mucous of the nose or the conjunctiva of the eye. If it is asthma, the bronchial mucous will react immediately. If a reaction takes place, the test result is positive.

Our Body
and Allergies

We have already discussed how an allergic reaction is produced in our bodies, and what provokes it.

Now we will explore more in depth the three elements of our body that are involved when it comes to triggering an allergic reaction. These elements are the immune system, our intestine, and our liver. They are fundamental pieces in the day-to-day function of the human body, and it is essential to keep them in optimum condition in order to avoid these types of problems, among other reasons.

The Immune System

It is the white knight of our organism, our personal army that defends us from foreign invaders.

It is composed of a vital set of cells and tissues that protect our bodies from foreign agents like bacteria, viruses, fungi, and certain chemicals. In normal conditions the immune system recognizes which of these substances are potentially dangerous and reacts in an efficient way to eliminate them.

Also, it has the capacity to recognize the cells that form parts of our bodies, and so avoids harming them when the defense mechanisms are put in place, only destroying the foreign agents in the body.

What organs form the immune system? The system of organs that form the immune system is called "the lymphatic system." They cause the growth, development, and release of antibodies or white blood cells called "lymphocytes."

The blood vessels and the lymphatic vessels also form an important part of the lymphocyte organs, as they are the mode of transport for the lymphocytes to many parts of the body, and from these parts to other areas. Each one of those lymphocyte organs plays an important role in the production and activation of the lymphocytes. They are the following:

- **Adenoids:** two glands located in the back of the nasal passage.
- **Appendix:** small tube attached to the large intestine.
- **Blood vessels:** arteries, veins, and capillaries through which blood travels.
- **Bone Marrow:** Soft grey tissue located in the bone cavities.
- **Lymph Nodes:** small bean-shaped organs that are found throughout the body and are connected by the lymphatic vessels.
- **Lymphatic Vessels:** a network of canals throughout the body that carries lymphocytes to the lymphoid organs and bloodstream.
- **Peyer's Patch:** lymphatic tissue in the small intestine.
- **Spleen:** organ the size of a fist located in the abdominal cavity.
- **Thymus:** two lobes that join in front of the trachea and behind the sternum.

How does it work? Every cell has its own characteristics that are accepted and recognized by the rest of the body. Because of this, when a foreign element, or antigen, enters our bodies, it immediately triggers an immune response that starts the production of antibodies, white blood cells charged with expelling or destroying the foreign element.

The defense is not just carried out in one of our organs, but is coordinated between the brain, glands, skin, bone marrow, hormones, and other messaging substances, and an enormous amount of antibodies.

When a foreign element enters the body, the antibodies make an analysis of its characteristics. Every antibody identifies one of these elements, attaches to it, and warns the phagocytes, another type of white blood cells that are in our blood. From this moment, the phagocytes begin to destroy the membrane of the foreign element with the help of enzymes.

In the case that the attack is on a virus or large numbers of germs, the defenders send messenger substances to other types of white blood cells and leukocytes to come to the rescue; these are our greatest defense. These include T lymphocytes (produced by the thymus) and B lymphocytes (produced by the marrow), which when paired with the offenders begin to reproduce in large quantities. The first destroy the enemy and the second transform to become antibodies or immunoglobulin G, which play a fundamental role in allergies if they later become specific immunoglobulins or IgE.

When everything is under control, other cells called "suppressors" appear, to calm the defenders, which sometimes begin to destroy healthy cells. If B lymphocytes don't control the situation, immune or allergic reaction is produced.

If the immune system wins the battle, the defenders register the facts collected from the elements that they attacked and archive them in their memories, so that before a new attack of these same germs, they can begin to produce the corresponding antibodies and in doing so fight the illness before it repeats itself. In the case of an allergen-triggered response, the reaction is identical, whereby each new exposure to the allergen provokes a response from the E immunoglobulins.

Types of Immunity. The immune system has many different responsibilities. As we have described, it not only provides protection against infection that comes from outside of our defense barriers, but it also adapts itself to provide immunity, as it registers the characteristics of infectious microorganisms from previous exposure. The grade and duration of the immune response depends on the type and quantity of antigen that it has combated and of the form in which this invades our body.

Natural immunity creates natural barriers in the body, like skin and protective substances in the mouth, the urinary tract, and the surface of the eye. Another type is made up of antibodies that are passed from mother to child.

Another type exists called "acquired immunity." This is developed with continued exposure to specific foreign microorganisms — toxins, strange tissues, or all of these — that fight allergens recognized by our immune system. One example of this is measles. Once we are exposed to measles or the measles vaccine, our immune system produces specific antibodies against it. When we are exposed to measles again, our immune system triggers the production of these specific antibodies against measles to combat the illness and keep us safe.

Immune Dysfunctions. When the immune system suffers a disruption in its different functions, three groups of ailments occur. In the first case, autoimmune diseases, the immune system can't distinguish its own cells from foreign ones, and the defense mechanisms harm tissues in the same person as if they were foreign elements. This is the case in many ailments, as in rheumatoid arthritis or multiple sclerosis.

The second group consists of immune deficiencies. Here the system doesn't function and the organism can't defend itself from infections, as in the case of AIDS.

And the third is in the case of allergies, which we'll focus on in the following pages.

Understanding Your Intestine

Maybe this will surprise you, but the intestine plays a fundamental role in the origin and development of allergies. There is a proven connection between both, despite the fact that in many cases, the person who suffers from allergies is not aware of it.

The majority of people believe that their intestine works like clockwork, but many specialists of natural medicine have taken this opportunity to prove that this is not the case. Just ask a couple of questions to begin to note irregularities in the intestinal track. The healthy goal of evacuating it once a day is not always achieved and problems can begin to develop, very subtly at first, but become compounded later. They do not usually cause discomfort and cramping pains, and for this, they can pass unnoticed. This does not lead to awareness of the importance of a healthy diet.

Intestinal problems do not only cause allergies, but can also cause illnesses such as gastrointestinal ulcers, inflammation of the large intestine, diverticulitis, bile discomfort and even intestinal cancer. Other problems exist that have to do with the function of our intestine, like migraines, acne, rheumatic pains, depression, or aggressiveness.

We will try to explain in simple terms the function of your digestive apparatus and how you have to treat it to maintain your health and not produce undesirable pains.

How does it work? Although it seems obvious, it is necessary to begin by saying that digestion begins in the mouth with chewing the food and salivating. This initial step is key, as insufficient chewing can cause discomfort later in its digestion. Therefore, it is necessary to eat slowly and to chew every bite a minimum of thirty times so that the food can make it to the stomach well-crushed and thoroughly covered in saliva.

After traveling through the esophagus, the food arrives in the stomach, which is a widening in the digestive tract. This two-quart capacity sack has a strong muscle in its entrance and one in its exit. Food arrives here to be processed during what is the only stop in the trip through the body. This stop does not have a determined length. There are quite indigestible foods like canned fish that can remain there for as many as eight hours.

The average time spent digesting food is more or less three hours when the stomach is dealing with light and balanced food.

In the stomach, the food proteins are predigested with the help of the enzyme pepsin, among others. This enzyme only acts as an environmental acid, to which the gastric juices of the stomach contribute and also kill bacteria.

After leaving the stomach, the predigested foods arrive in the small intestine, and it is here where digestion really begins, that is to say, the assimilation of the nutrients from the food that we have eaten three hours before. The small intestine is a tube about twenty feet long in the abdominal cavity, folded tightly. Its inside is covered in an intestinal mucous that absorbs nutrients. To augment this absorption, the lining of the tube has protrusions on it in the shape of fingers whose surface is covered in hairs. This form enormously multiplies its functions. The absorbed nutrients are transported through the body by the capillaries and the central lymphatic vessels.

Nevertheless, the process is more complicated than it seems. Foods need to be broken down into smaller elements or amino acids for our body to truly assimilate the nutrients. The cells and glands in the intestinal mucous and the pancreas produce digestive juices and begin hydrolysis (breaking down chemical bonds with water molecules) of fats, carbohydrates, and proteins in their smaller components. Along with bile, which is produced by the liver and is stored in the vesicles, it contributes to the digestion of fats.

On the wall of the small intestine are many long muscular fibers that produce small constant oscillating movements to help facilitate thorough mixing of the food pulp. There are other muscular fibers that transport the content of the large intestine through other undulating contractions.

Next, the food arrives in the large intestine or colon, which is five feet long and has another important function for our body: it collects electrolytes, vitamins, and water from the food pulp so that the body does not lose it. We are talking about more than one-and-a-half gallons of digestive juices that our body wouldn't absorb any other way. Also, the colon houses beneficial bacteria (*lactobacillus acidophilus* and *bifidus*) that play a vital role in our health and in the organisms of allergic people. Only in the last few years have we learned that we are able to digest the cells that have not been decomposed well by the digestive juices and produce vitamins that are fundamental to our health. These bacteria are finally distributed in the small intestine and the large intestine and form the intestinal mucous. But, also, they form a compact layer that covers the internal wall and they train the lymphatic tissue of defense of our organism to fight against pathogens. Seventy percent of the lymphatic tissue in the digestive tract is found in the intestinal wall.

The intestinal mucous is composed of one single layer of cells that is renewed every two days. Only twenty-five thousandths of a millimeter separate the content of the intestine from the bloodstream. Given the extreme thinness of the intestinal wall, your body is vulnerable to whatever enters the intestine and it depends on the appropriate selection of what should or should not enter the bloodstream or lymphatic system. Among the group of substances that should not pass through the intestinal wall are allergens. Because of this, it is important to maintain optimal conditions in your digestive track.

Response to the aggressions. Our digestive system is our fountain of energy. Its structure and function are very complex and it is not difficult to disrupt its equilibrium, causing serious consequences that can be detrimental to our health. Even though it is resistant and tolerates our bad eating habits, there comes a moment when it cannot respond the way we need it to and illness occurs as a result.

We are the only ones responsible for this unbalance. Eating too fast, on-the-go, and poorly are not the best ways to eat, but they are what often prevail in our busy day-to-day lives. We don't refrain from binge eating and punishing our digestive systems with too much rich, fatty food. This way of eating results in an overload and in exhaustion of our pancreas, and leaves our food incompletely digested.

If a food isn't digested properly it ferments or rots in the body. This process provokes the formation of annoying gases and the sensation of fullness, or indigestion. Even though a majority of the gases are eliminated, the blood also absorbs a small percentage through the intestinal wall and it overloads the liver. They are responsible for migraine, depression, or torpor. Because of this, it is also important to have our livers, the laboratory of our bodies, in optimal conditions.

When the pancreas cannot function at full capacity, digestion is carried out with a deficit of pancreatic juices, without which the nutrients cannot break down thoroughly in the small intestine.

As if all this were not enough, as we ingest refined products full of pesticides, this produces degradation in the intestinal environment. This is aggravated by the consumption of alcohol and white sugar.

Even though this seems like an apocalyptic situation, it occurs more often than we think.

All these factors contribute to a chronic irritation of the intestinal mucous, an inflammation of the intestinal walls, the conducts of the intestinal walls, the conducts of the bile vesicles, and the pancreas, resulting in poor digestion and inadequate absorption of nutrients essential to our health.

When the intestinal environment is in bad condition, the large allergenic proteins can begin to penetrate our body because there is not a consistent barrier that stops them, as the flora and intestinal mucous is degraded. In a healthy intestine, proteins cannot pass through the intestinal lining. Instead they are broken down and only amino acids are allowed to pass, which are the result of the unfolding of the proteins and which our bodies can absorb with no problem.

Foods like carbohydrates and sugar produce alcohol in an intestine with damaged flora because they ferment. The intestinal environment can barely control the scarce beneficial bacteria and produces a proliferation of fungus.

The beneficial bacteria train our immune system in the fight against infection and undesirable microorganisms, and their shortage holds a serious danger for our physical and psychological equilibrium.

What can influence the state of our intestinal mucous?

When the intestinal walls are inflamed, a putrefaction of the foods results, and harmful substances attack the intestinal walls. Also, it can influence an insufficient diet in protective substances, which augments the permeability of our intestine and produces what is called "intestinal hyperpermeability." Among the most common cases the following stand out:

- **Excess of animal fats.** Saturated animal fats, including butter, are rich in butyric acid, an element that degrades vitamin F (polyunsaturated fatty acids) and permeates the intestinal wall. Also, an excess of fats and fried foods can provoke an excessive secretion of bile that damages the intestinal wall.

- **Excess of animal protein.** Vegetables just ferment in the gut, but animal-based foods rot. You can tell from the language which type of food better suits our bodies.

- **Unhealthy diet.** A diet rich in vegetables, whole grains, legumes, and seaweed helps with the development of beneficial intestinal bacteria, which also fight against harmful bacteria like Escherichia Coli and fungi like candida. These harmful bacteria are caused by an excess of meat products and can create damage to the intestinal mucous.

- **Medicines.** Antibiotics, which damage beneficial intestinal flora; aspirins, which are corrosive to the digestive mucous (because of this, they shouldn't be taken on an empty stomach); steroids; and food additives have many negative effects in the mucous.

- **Irritants to the intestinal mucous:** Coffee, sugar, alcohol, cacao, tobacco, and certain spices.

- **Food Intolerances.** Cause fermentation of several nutrients that can't be digested correctly (lactose, gluten, casein, etc) and their by-products (among others, alcohol) irritate the mucous.

- **Deficit of polyunsaturated fatty acids (omega 3 and omega 6).** These fatty acids aid in elasticity and adaptability in the intestinal cellular membranes, which also influence the level of permeability of the mucous. As this is regenerated often, it is necessary to replenish these nutrients daily.

- **Diet lacking in carotenes and/or vitamins.** Carotenes are the precursors to vitamin A, essential to preserving the well-being of skin and mucous. Vitamin E (antioxidant of fats and protector of cellular membranes) and vitamin C (antioxidant and necessary for the maintenance of conjunctive tissue) are also important. All of these can be obtained through fruits and vegetables.

You have the solution. Many people in the western world who are victims of stress and of a diet rich in sugar and processed foods have intestinal problems. These problems are not solved by taking medicine.

If it is true that it takes years to damage the intestinal flora, the fact remains that it requires sacrifice and willpower by each of us to reestablish the equilibrium in our digestive system. You cannot succeed in healing the intestine and restore the flora in two weeks if it has been mistreated for several years. Nevertheless, from here on out, we encourage you to do so with the assessment of a medical professional. It is possible that it will take a few months, but there will be great health benefits, and we are not referring only to allergies.

To start, you should eat whole, natural foods, and completely cut out sugar, white flour, alcohol, and pork. In the chapter **Allergic Diseases: Natural Solutions**, we give some basic guidelines to help you follow a healthy and balanced diet.

It is necessary that you make gradual changes to your diet. We don't recommend that you make a drastic or sudden change since foods like raw vegetables or grains can be difficult to digest for an intestine with problems. The final goal is a highly nutritious diet that supports your body for a great function, including the immune system. But this won't be fixed immediately. Meanwhile, chew thoroughly and wait about four hours between meals to avoid overloading your stomach and intestines.

In addition to changing your diet, your specialist can help you renew your intestinal flora with natural products and prescribe, after examining a stool sample, natural drugs to kill fungi and protozoa.

It is a slow process, but restoring your intestinal flora is crucial to restoring your health.

COLON THERAPY

One method that therapists use to remove the residue of fermented and rotten food in your intestine is colon hydrotherapy or colon therapy. If we eat poorly or suffer from constipation, evacuation can be incomplete or difficult and toxins can accumulate in our bodies, creating serious problems.

Colon therapy uses smooth controlled currents of water that is pumped into the initial portion of the large intestine, cleaning heavy particles of accumulated debris. Even a gentle abdominal massage and pressing certain points can help eliminate waste. The water that is used is at a temperature of about 100°F. It also contains salt and an infusion of herbs that reduce the swelling of your intestinal wall and help drain your liver.

This therapy has been practiced for thousands of years in Western countries. The fact that you don't need to take medicine to help solve the problem is one of its benefits, and it increases muscle tone so as to facilitate the peristaltic action and increase the absorption of nutrients while minimizing toxic waste elements.

THE INTESTINE AND MILK PRODUCTS

In the section on food allergies this book will offer comprehensive information on dairy products and their impact on the organisms that produce allergies and those that are responsible for food intolerance.

Even if your body can tolerate these foods, nutrition experts do not recommend them at all, because they contain a high percentage of chemicals and drugs that pollute our body. The milk that is marketed today has nothing to do with the fresh milk our parents and grandparents used to drink, and is one of the most processed products in the world.

In addition, dairy products promote the production of mucous, so it is recommended to decrease their consumption to improve this symptom in people with colds or respiratory allergies.

Some studies claim that one of the causes of excessive mucous is the pH level in dairy products like yogurt, while other sources point to the proteins found in cow's milk, like casein, as the cause. Although the direct relationship between dairy and increased mucous production is not known, it is certain that a moderate or restricted presence of dairy products in your diet decreases the amount of mucous significantly. This clears up nasal congestion and facilitates easier breathing.

Reducing dairy intake is recommended even when there are no physical problems, as the excess mucous can clog membranes and facilitate the onset of disease. Specialists in natural medicine claim that dairy products are responsible for conditions such as hay fever, asthma, bronchitis, sinusitis, colds, runny noses, and ear infections. In general, they are also the main cause of allergies. Removing dairy from your diet for just a few months if you have any of these conditions will lead to improvements.

SUGAR

Nowadays, levels of sugar consumption in Western society are very high. However, this was not the case just a few decades ago. Then, our supply of glucose came from grains and simple sugars in fruit, which contain carbohydrates that are absorbed slowly into our systems. However, today we eat refined white sugar, which has poor consequences on our health.

Sugar is high in calories, and can cause an imbalance in our metabolism. Like milk and dairy, it also causes the body to produce excess mucous. Excessive drinking can overwork the liver, which is responsible for regulating the level of blood sugar and also affects the activity of white blood cells and leukocytes by reducing their antimicrobial capacity. This can cause diabetes, obesity, and vascular problems, and also promotes demineralization in our body and negatively affects our energy, as it tends to balance certain chemical elements in our body such as calcium, iron, phosphorus, and B vitamins.

Refined sugar only provides empty calories and causes us to run out of energy quickly.

Consuming any amount of refined sugar is not recommended for anyone, but still less for people with allergies or excess mucous.

The Role of the Liver

Allergies are closely related to the liver, not only the immune system or the bowel. Liver function is also a decisive factor in the presence of allergies.

The liver is the second largest organ in our body and in some ways the most complex. It has been nicknamed the "laboratory of the body" and is responsible for filtering out toxins. These toxic substances come from the intestine primarily, but can reach any part of the body. The liver is the great purifier of our blood and it uses many tools to do its job: hormones, clotting factors, and cholesterol for the proper functioning of bile, among others.

If excess toxic substances are circulating in our body, the kidneys, intestine, and lungs remove them naturally. If it is overloaded with toxins, the liver cannot process them correctly, and this results in rhinitis, excess mucous inflammation, rashes, and more.

Excess toxins come from an unbalanced diet with large amounts of chemical elements in foods, excessive consumption of fats and sugars, environmental pollution, lack of rest, or states of nervousness or stress; in short, toxins come from an unhealthy lifestyle.

The status of the liver is also addressed in traditional Chinese medicine, which defines the load on the liver as an excess of yang. Symptoms of stress on the liver are redness and itching, and one of the most affected elements is the metal element, which corresponds to the lungs and large intestine. The consequences of these symptoms are allergies, especially rhinitis and conjunctivitis.

From the point of view of this medicine, the main cause of excess yang in the liver is usually related to diet. Yang foods include animal products, foods that contain a high amount of salt, overly cooked foods, foods high in sugar such as soft drinks, sweets, and alcohol. Consuming a "yang-heavy" diet is bad for our bodies.

The views are different but the conclusions are the same: you have to take care of your liver. Lead an orderly life, get plenty of sleep, avoid stress, and be very careful of your diet.

Can You Cure Allergies?

Everyone who suffers from allergies asks this question, and the answer seems uncertain in many cases.

Allergy sufferers often do not understand what is happening and come to believe that they have brought this chronic disease upon themselves. They find it difficult to understand that substances that do not hurt other people are somehow harmful to them. The medical explanation is often of little comfort, because while it is known that allergens trigger an allergic reaction, it is harder to understand how the reaction is caused by something as seemingly harmless as pollen.

Conventional medicine says that allergies cannot be cured, and instead focuses on relieving the uncomfortable symptoms. In some very specific cases, such as the response to a single allergen, a vaccine-based therapy can be performed that "reprograms" our immune system, deactivating the excessive immune response. But it is uncommon to be allergic to one single allergen, let alone trace the reaction back to that specific allergen. Some people are sensitive to cold, dust, food, and medicine at once, for example. Patients often make many visits to specialists and undergo several treatments with poor results.

In many cases, the disappointment in conventional treatments leads the patient and personal physician to consider a new approach. Filled with mistrust after successive disappointments, they turn to the homeopath, acupuncturist, or naturopath with the hope that these therapies will help them to live without allergies.

Holistic medicine has a different concept of disease from conventional medicine and the main focus is not on the disease but the patient. The goal is to return the body and mind to health without the use of chemical substances that disrupt our organism's balance and produce unwanted side effects. A healthy diet of natural foods is always recommended in tandem with personalized treatments that are designed to harmonize and modify the physical and emotional functions of the patient and strengthen the immune system.

These methods help to fix the patient's problems, but there is no doubt that in the case of anaphylactic shock or a severe asthma attack requiring emergency medical care, administration of anti-inflammatories is necessary to stop a process that may have fatal consequences.

Anyone who thinks that an allergy should only be treated for symptoms is incorrect. The consequences of a prolonged treatment with anti-allergy drugs such as corticosteroids or antihistamines are harmful to the rest of the body and do not cure the allergy. They only relieve your symptoms. The medicine's mechanistic approach, that is, conventional medicine, generates disappointment in many patients.

Holistic medicine instead seeks to heal the body completely, to help you restore balance. A balanced body is a healthy body. This balance can be achieved through attention to several factors: treatment, diet, exercise, and relaxation. And the ultimate goal is you.

To take advantage of this you must get medical guidance. However, that is not enough. It is also essential for you to take responsibility for yourself and your health. If you choose to pursue natural treatments, you should not only avoid the allergen causing your health problems, but it is also imperative that you change your eating and living habits, and strictly follow your specialist's instructions. Then you will be able to work together on this important journey toward your recovery.

When Should You Consult a Doctor?

Although you believe that the decision to choose a natural treatment to overcome your allergy is the healthiest approach, sometimes a serious situation occurs that requires urgent medical attention. In this case, it is necessary that you go to the hospital as soon as possible for medical treatment.

If you have a very serious allergy, there are also some medications such as a bronchodilator, which can save your life, and it would be reckless (and possibly dangerous) to give up this option just because you're otherwise following a natural method of treatment. Severe symptoms require medical attention.

However, not all allergic reactions require that level of urgent care. The following are situations when you should go to the doctor without fail:

- **If your skin suddenly becomes blotchy, along with redness and itching**, you may also have tachycardia (rapid heart rate). In this case, chances are you're facing an anaphylactic shock, which is the most dangerous allergic reaction. Anaphylactic shock requires urgent medical treatment because it can be fatal.
- **If breathing is difficult or labored, with the sensation of drowning,** this may be an acute asthma attack, a severe allergic reaction or a heart attack. This kind of attack requires urgent medical treatment.
- **If you feel intestinal or stomach pain, diarrhea, or vomiting,** this could be due to a severe food allergy or food poisoning. It is necessary that you go to the doctor as soon as possible.

Conventional Medical Treatment

Conventional medicine treats allergies with a range of drugs, which can help solve the patient's problems. The symptoms are alleviated, and life becomes more bearable. However, these drugs often come with side effects that are as bad as the previous symptoms.

While these inevitable side effects are not easy to manage, it is important to remember that in the case of a severe allergy, these drugs can save your life in an emergency.

As in every situation, there is nothing absolutely good or absolutely bad. We advocate a holistic approach to treat your allergies, try to correct the source of your ailment, and balance your body so that you can overcome your allergies. However, you are responsible for your life and your health, and your primary concern should be to choose the method that best suits the way you think and live.

If you decide to choose a conventional drug treatment, do so under supervision of an expert allergist.

Below, we will explain the different types of drugs that are prescribed to treat allergy symptoms.

Antihistamines. Our body releases histamine in the presence of allergens during an allergic reaction. Histamine causes swelling, redness, and itching, and may be released in both mucous membranes and skin.

To help mediate this powerful substance, there are drugs that block mast cells or histamine receptors and supersede the itchy and inflamed effects. The drugs work for a short duration and must be taken daily, as they only act as histamine blockers.

They are primarily used to relieve or prevent the symptoms of allergic rhinitis, and are marketed as tablets, capsules, liquids, or injections. They can be purchased with or without prescription, although we recommend that you only take them with a prescription from your physician.

Antihistamines are divided into sedatives, which often cause drowsiness and an increase in appetite. The active ingredients Are: ebastine, loratadine, cetirizine, azelastine, and levocabastine.

Antihistamines may provoke dry mouth, difficulty urinating, constipation, irritability, and trouble sleeping. Other side effects that may occur with the use of antihistamines include cardiovascular, gastrointestinal, and respiratory reactions, and rarely hematological, neurological, or genitourinary reactions.

Anti-inflammatory agents. These potent drugs are used to treat acute symptoms of inflammation, one of the major drawbacks of allergies that can affect the skin; eczema; allergic rhinitis; ocular conjunctiva; and the bronchi in cases of asthma. Symptoms can range from mild to very severe and this scale depends on the dose for each individual patient, especially in cases of respiratory inflammation or asthma. It is therefore very important to have your doctor decide the treatment, its duration, and what dosage you should take.

Below, we list the anti-inflammatory agents that are used most frequently:

TOPICAL NASAL STEROIDS

These most often come in the form of drops that are inhaled through the nose to reduce nasal congestion and relieve associated symptoms, especially in allergic rhinitis. They are also sold in tablets, although these do not act directly on the area in question so their action is not as fast and the required dose is higher.

This medication causes contraction of the blood vessels in the nose, which eliminates the nasal congestion, sneezing,

NATURAL TREATMENT OF ALLERGIES

and dripping. You can purchase them with or without a prescription.

These pills can be taken in conjunction with an antihistamine for stronger results. While there are benefits to this, the combination results in side effects like nervousness, insomnia, and increased blood pressure.

The active ingredients are anti-inflammatory glucocorticoids fluticasone and budesonide. Although they are immediately effective, the relief is compounded if you take them a few times daily as recommended by your allergist.

However, if you abuse these drugs, you can dry out the inside of your nose and provoke epitasis or nosebleeds.

In addition, taking them over a long period of time can cause rebound rhinitis. The abuse of these drugs causes congestion that is not due to an allergic reaction, but to a dependency on the medication.

CORTICOSTEROIDS

Corticosteroids are a very effective anti-inflammatory steroid and have nothing to do with anabolic steroids, which some athletes use to improve their performance and muscle mass.

They are found in the typical asthma inhaler that people carry, and should always carry, to make sure you have treatment during an attack.

These drugs are also taken in pill or liquid form, and can even be injected.

Among the minor side effects of using corticosteroid inhalers are frequent hoarseness, and thrush infection caused by a fungus in the mouth and throat. Its incidence is lower if you rinse your mouth with water, gargle, and spit out drug residues after use.

It also has serious side effects. For example, although the benefits are great, prolonged use in children has been shown to potentially stunt or slow their growth.

Steroids and Children

The powerful anti-inflammatory effects of steroids make them one of the best weapons in an allergist's arsenal to treat childhood asthma and allergic rhinitis in children, but they can cause a delay in children's bone growth if used in large doses over long periods of time.

The reason for this effect is that steroids act on the cartilage growth. Cartilage acts as a cushion in between bones, and is about seven millimeters thick. As the child grows, the cartilage slowly ossifies, that is, progressively hardens while the bone forms because of the accumulation of minerals, especially calcium. This process usually ends after about twenty years, when it is considered that the person has completed their growth period.

However, this dangerous side effect is directly related to the methods of administration of the drug, and it is not common in the case of inhaler use. These changes in growth have occurred when corticosteroids were administered orally (tablets) or injection (parenteral), and over an extended period of time.

In the case of children, it is advisable to take corticosteroids through a nasal or bronchial inhaler. This almost entirely avoids the risk of affecting the rate of growth, while preventing major or fatal allergic reactions.

The short-term adverse effects in adults are a slight weight gain, increased appetite, menstrual irregularities, cramps, heartburn, and indigestion. These side effects usually go away quickly once the patient stops taking the corticosteroids. However, they can also affect the immune system and fluid retention, so a doctor should always prescribe them. In addition, diabetics cannot take them because they increase blood sugar, and neither can those who have hypertension as the corticosteroids increase blood pressure.

MAST CELL STABILIZERS

These medicines are NSAIDs (non-steroidal anti-inflammatory drugs). Their main action is to reduce inflammation and prevent the release of histamine from mast cells. They are mostly used in cases of allergic rhinitis and conjunctivitis.

Cromolyn, nedocromil, and lodoxamina are common NSAIDs and are either inhaled, or taken in the form of eye drops to combat allergic conjunctivitis.

You may have to take it several times a day as directed by your doctor, and it may take up to two weeks to get the full results. Its benefits are more preventative than anything, and they are not very potent drugs. Their common side effects are sneezing and itchy, burning, or watery eyes.

ANTILEUKOTRINES

Leukotrines are chemical elements that produce many of the cells that are linked to inflammation of the airways. They increase inflammation in the body, tighten the muscles in the airways, and increase leakage of blood vessels in the respiratory tract.

They are a relatively new type of medication to help control the symptoms of persistent asthma by preventing the narrowing of the airways and reducing fluid in the lungs.

One of these medicines has also been approved to treat allergic rhinitis.

BRONCHODILATORS

Bronchodilators help open the airway and relieve coughs, wheezing, and difficulty breathing.

They are called "rescue medications" and are administered in acute asthma attacks. They are fast-acting and used as needed as symptoms occur. There are other bronchodilators that need to act slower and are prescribed for maintenance or daily use to help control outbreaks. Below are several types of bronchodilators:

- **Beta agonists.** These medications relax the bronchial tube muscles.

  There are two kinds. Fast-acting drugs that cause immediate relief, such as albuterol, can be inhaled, taken in pill or liquid form, or injected. Those of prolonged action are used for long-term control of asthma, and are often prescribed salmeterol or formoterol. Side effects include tachycardia, nervousness, insomnia, and, sometimes headaches.

- **Theophylline.** It can be administered in tablets, capsules, or intravenous injections. If you are prescribed this medication, you will need to monitor your blood. Side effects include headaches, palpitations, and digestive disturbances.
- **Anticholinergics.** They can be taken alone or in combination with beta-agonist bronchodilators. They are administered as inhalers, pills, liquids, or injections.

Among them is ipratropium, which is used to treat asthma and provides quick relief.

Its side effects are coughing and headaches.

Omalizumab. This new drug was first prescribed in 2003 in the United States and the European Union approved it in late 2005.

It is considered by many allergists to be one of the most important achievements that occurred in the last decade in the fight against asthma, but it is only prescribed to adults and children over twelve years old.

Omalizumab is recommended for patients with severe persistent allergic asthma. Technically, it is a therapeutic monoclonal antibody that binds in a specific manner and blocks immunoglobulin E, the immunoglobulin responsible for inflammation that causes allergic diseases.

It is administered through subcutaneous injections every two to four weeks. But it should be prescribed only to patients with moderate to severe persistent allergic asthma who have not had good results with traditional therapy. It is also administered in cases where inhaled or oral steroids cause the patient to suffer significant side effects. It is also used in the case of those requiring urgent care in hospitals due to an asthma attack or significant daily problems.

Immunotherapy or vaccines. When drugs do not work, or it is impossible for the patient to avoid contact with certain allergens, you can use vaccines or immunotherapy. These methods are used most commonly in the case of mites, mold, pollen, insect bites, or pet allergies.

This treatment is administered over the course of several years to an allergic patient who suffers bad allergic reactions. The dosage is increased slowly in order to reach the patient's tolerance without causing an allergic reaction.

The patient is able to build a tolerance against the allergen because the body begins to produce protective antibodies in response to the vaccine. It also changes the cells of the immune system that regulate the allergic reactions, mainly in T lymphocytes.

This therapy may temporarily cure the allergy in the case of several allergens. You can even get to permanently cure one or two of them.

The allergy shots work well when treating allergic rhinitis, allergic conjunctivitis, allergies to bee stings, and some drug allergies. In some people, they can also improve the symptoms of asthma. This treatment has a minimum duration of one year. It begins with one or two weekly shots over six months containing a small amount of extract with the lowest possible concentration of the drug. The solution is gradually increased and the administration times are lengthened. The entire treatment can take three to five years depending on the patient's sensitivity. Drugs are often prescribed while the vaccines are administered to help relieve any allergy symptoms, which will decrease as the vaccines take effect.

The new generation of vaccines available today only uses a portion of the protein allergen instead of the entire protein. These changes have ensured that their effectiveness in desensitization is very high.

However, not everyone can be vaccinated. This treatment is not recommended for people who suffer from serious asthma or heart problems, are pregnant, or are less than five years old.

Although generally considered a safe treatment, vaccinations also carry some risks. Because they contain small amounts of allergen, the patient could have an allergic reaction to the vaccine itself, such as swelling at the site where the vaccine is given. However, there can also be more dangerous reactions, such as anaphylactic shock. Although this kind of reaction is rare, you should always consult an allergist to make sure the dosage of allergens is accurate.

Natural Treatment of Allergies

The tools provided to cope with, and perhaps cure, allergies through conventional medicine do not attack the root of the problem. Your body is a well-oiled machine and if one piece does not work, the whole system is thrown off. When it comes to allergies, however, the origin of the flaw in the immune system is difficult to pinpoint, and conventional medicine only provides palliative solutions to relieve allergy symptoms, and they often cause side effects.

Natural allergy treatment does not explain the origin of our immune system's dysfunction. As when pursuing a treatment through conventional medicine, the patient is advised to stay away from the allergen or allergens in question, but a natural treatment differs in its initial approach. For natural therapies, our body and mind are treated as a single unit, and the treatments seek to achieve balance between the two. These therapies provide different tools to solve our health problems: a healthy lifestyle and diet, and a natural treatment without side effects.

The goal is to return the body to normal, in the hopes that the immune system will stop overreacting to harmless substances. When our body and our mind are in perfect balance, they function together like clockwork.

This natural approach opens the door to a life full of hope, and provides solutions that cannot be achieved through conventional treatment. A healthy diet, a more relaxed pace of life, plenty of rest, herbal treatments, homeopathy, and other useful therapies will help you regenerate your body and balance your immune system.

Using a variety of methods will help you fine-tune your body and relieve stress. If you feed your body with nutritious foods, avoiding refined products and chemical additives, if your mind provides a peaceful space for you to reflect on your day, if your body is not subjected to the side effects of drugs, you have great potential to free yourself from the allergy that is affecting your life.

In the chapter **Allergic Diseases: Natural Solutions**, we will describe several diets that can help you begin to heal.

Common Allergens:
How to Combat
Their Effects

Allergens are, for most people, harmless particles that are present in the air we breathe, what we eat, and what we touch. However, for unknown reasons, these particles cause allergic reactions in some individuals.

There are many types of allergens. Many are proteins, although there are also intolerances and allergies to metals, chemical additives, and irritants such as solvents, cigarette smoke, and pollution.

In this section we describe the most common allergens and irritants and how you can avoid them.

Pollen

These plant proteins trigger seasonal allergies, which are usually manifested as allergic rhinitis, extrinsic asthma, allergic conjunctivitis, depression, discomfort, or fatigue. Pollen allergies usually occur in young people, especially teenagers, but they can get better later in life.

But what is pollen? Pollen is the male germ cell of flowering plants, a particle that is natural and necessary for the reproduction of many plant species. This complex particle contains over twelve different substances to which the mucous membranes of an allergic person can respond with hay fever or a pollen allergy.

Species that usually cause allergies are varied and called "wind-pollinated plants." Their times of pollination occur throughout the year.

The question that arises when you begin to study cases of pollen allergies is the following: Why is there a higher proportion of people allergic to pollen in cities than in rural areas? The former seems contradictory, since there is a larger concentration of pollen in rural areas than in cities, because there are more trees and other plant life. However, numerous studies have shown that pollen floating in the urban air contains a dangerous layer of adhered environmental contaminants like carbon dioxide emitted by the exhaust from the thousands of vehicles in cities, together with the emissions from heaters and the scarcity of green areas. This factor makes the pollen particle a small but powerful "allergic bomb" that is a more potent irritant than the pollen you breathe in the streets of a small town or farm. Air pollution has caused pollen to become increasingly allergenic and trigger more reactions in sensitive people. Other studies suggest that pollen from a polluted environment can cause a more virulent immune response than that from a clean atmosphere. As we cannot always up and move to the country, no matter how much we may want to, here are some guidelines for living with a pollen allergy in an urban area.

Avoid pollen as much as possible: keep your environment clean to keep your body clean.

Tree pollen. There are several different pollination periods for trees. If you suffer from hay fever, you will likely suffer from allergic reactions from February through April due to pollen from trees like banana, pine, birch, beech, poplar, hazel, and alder. From October to March, you could also suffer from a cypress pollen allergy.

If you have an allergy to tree pollen, eating certain fruits like apples, peaches, pears, cherries, and grapes can also trigger a reaction.

Fortunately, in the case of pollen from trees, no cross-reactions usually occur, so if you are allergic to banana trees, you will not also be allergic to birch trees, for example. While these allergies are triggered by certain kinds of trees, pollen can be transported tens of miles by the wind, so you can have an allergic response while not in a pine forest or surrounded by banana trees.

Roses will not give you allergies

Pollen allergies only occur in species that pollinate through the air like certain flowers and leafy plants. However, brightly colored flowers with pungent aromas use insects as a transport medium for pollen. The reason for this coloring and perfume is to attract insects like bees, in order to maximize the chances of pollination.

So it is safe to give someone a bouquet of roses, though breathing in deeply may trigger a reaction if their mucous is already inflamed, causing it to react to minimum stimulus.

Pollen from grasses. If you suffer from allergies during May or September it is likely that your allergies are triggered by grass pollen. This plant family is comprised of seven genera and consists of about twelve thousand species. This makes them very difficult to avoid. In fact, grasses are estimated to account for 20 percent of the plant world. These include grasses like hay or alfalfa, and grains such as wheat, barley, rye, rice, or sugar cane, just to name a few. If freshly cut grass makes you sneeze, this could perhaps be hay fever, which is the name given to allergic rhinitis, although it is not caused by hay.

There are many common cross-reactions among types of grasses.

As there are so many species, it is likely that your allergy could continue for ten months a year, with a peak season between May and July. There is a strong correlation between rainfall and the amount of pollen present in the air. It has been found that there is a higher concentration of grass pollen in areas with heavy rain between October and March than in areas with dry winters.

Pollen from herbs. If you suffer from allergies from August to October, this can mean you have an autumnal allergy caused by pollen from plants like parietaria, ragweed, mugwort, and plantain. This allergy is usually crossed with reactions to parsley, pepper, mustard, cinnamon, cumin, dill, and nutmeg.

Wherever we are, whether in the city or in the countryside, the air will have more or less elevated pollen concentrations. This can make the daily lives of people with hay fever very difficult, but there are some steps that can offer some relief or prevent allergic crisis.

If you are allergic to pollen you should keep the doors and windows of your home closed, especially during seasons when plants are pollinating. It is recommended that you use an air conditioner to circulate the air in your home and to filter out the pollen particles. However, make sure the equipment is properly fitted with special filters to keep out the smaller particles.

Similarly, you should keep car windows closed while you are driving, and you should avoid riding a motorcycle or bicycle. If you don't want to give up cycling, make sure to wear sunglasses to protect your eyes, and a mask that covers your mouth and nose to help avoid breathing in pollution.

Flowers open early in the morning and release pollen. As the temperature rises during the day, the pollen rises with the heat.

As the earth's surface cools, convection currents cease and the pollen falls. If you exercise outdoors, you should avoid going out between five and ten in the morning and seven and ten in the evening. During these periods the amount of pollen in the atmosphere is higher, especially on sunny or windy days.

In rural areas, the pollen often "falls" earlier during the day than in the city, where the polluted air takes longer to cool down. This can take until about two in the morning.

This can explain rhinitis attacks or asthma in the middle of the night, especially if you sleep with the windows open.

For the same reason, you should avoid going out to the countryside during seasons when the pollen concentration is higher. The newspapers and television often report the daily pollen concentrations, especially in the spring.

You should also not dry clothes outside on those days and wear sunglasses to protect your eyes from exposure to pollen.

On rainy days the atmosphere is clean and pollen is deposited on the ground, making it ideal to take a walk if you suffer from allergies. If you decide to go out on windy or very sunny days, this can irritate the bronchi and cause sneezing. It is also advisable to consider the weather and environmental factors when choosing a travel destination so as to avoid having an attack that could ruin your vacation.

If you have outdoor pets that spend time on the patio, in the garden, or on the street, keep in mind that their fur will subsequently carry pollen into your home. Do not touch your pets when they first come back in the house, and brush them thoroughly to remove the pollen. If you suffer from allergies, however, ask someone else to do the brushing.

It is also important that you brush off your coat and hair before you reenter your home, and take a shower to get rid of any pollen that may have stuck to your skin or hair.

One last caution may seem extreme, but it is very useful — cover the bed, sofa, or desk with a sheet if you are not using them. Very carefully remove the sheet and wash it when you need access to this furniture.

When choosing a vacation spot, pick places near the sea or high in the mountains, where pollen concentrations tend to be much lower. Avoid valleys and forested areas, as they are pollen traps.

Dust Mites

In addition to pollen, dust mites are another major allergen. It is very common to hear that people are allergic to dust. However, what's responsible for the allergic reaction is not dust particles, but the small bugs that live in them: mites.

Dust in the home consists of small particles of plant and animal material. While this can be an irritant, more irritating still are the microscopic creatures that thrive on these particles. If you are allergic to the perennial droppings of these mites, you will suffer reactions frequently.

We may think that our home is immaculate and that there is not a speck of dust anywhere. But that is not true. We can do our best, dusting with a rag or a brush, but instead of removing the dust we end up simply redistributing it on our floors, furniture, drapes, and carpets.

Mites are found throughout the house. They thrive in certain environments and need heat and high humidity to survive. If you keep your home well ventilated and your vacuum cleaner has an anti-mite filter, you can manage and control the mites.

These troublesome tenants prefer to live in stuffed animals, the sofas, pillows, and beds. These places are warm and moist, providing a comfortable environment and plenty of food. They feed on fungi and the small particles of skin that we shed every day. An adult sheds an average of a quarter ounce of skin every day, which is enough material to feed a million mites.

And we're not talking about a high temperature. In fact, they survive between sixty and eighty degrees Fahrenheit, with an optimum temperature of seventy-five degrees, and an ideal humidity level of 80 percent. These conditions are optimal between May and October. However, they are still in our home the rest of the year as protonymphs or eggs, waiting to have better conditions in which to thrive again.

The mites cause allergies by direct aspiration of their droppings, and a single dust mite can produce up to one hundred times the weight of his body in waste during its lifetime. Most of the mites die when the humidity or temperature becomes extreme, but leave the waste. These droppings are very small, but heavy, and do not float in the air. This makes an air conditioner or air purifier ineffective, as the droppings settle on surfaces like furniture or bedding, where they can be directly inhaled, as by a child sleeping with a stuffed animal. Also that is the reason why those who are allergic to mites may have an attack when they get up or go to bed.

Try not to obsess over getting rid of mites completely, as they are so ubiquitous. Though you can thoroughly clean your house, your clothes and shoes will bring mites back in. Do your best and don't become discouraged.

What are mites?

Mites are not insects but arthropods as they have eight legs instead of six, like spiders. There are at least thirteen species of dust mites and all are well adapted to the environment of your home.

These primitive creatures do not have a developed respiratory system or eyes, and pass their short lives moving, eating, playing, and producing waste. The life cycle of a mite has several stages, from egg to adult. Females can lay about a hundred eggs during their lifetimes. Mites take two to five weeks to develop from egg to adult, depending on the species, and adults then live for two to four months.

The species that most commonly causes allergies is called *Dermatophagoides* (mainly *pteronyssinuss* and *farinae*).

Symptoms of an allergy to dust mites may include congestion or runny nose with bursts of sneezing (particularly in the morning), itchy and watery eyes, coughing, and wheezing.

How to eliminate mites from your home. It is not possible to completely eliminate mites from your life unless you live in the desert or on the North or South Pole, but you can take effective action against them and drastically improve your quality of life.

Although your home looks clean, it will always provide shelter to these microscopic tenants, but you can greatly reduce their numbers by taking action. While you cannot entirely eliminate them, getting rid of the majority of them will mean a significant improvement in your allergy symptoms.

Studies show that mites live better and in greater quantity in bedrooms. So let's start with directions on how to effectively attack them in your room.

Mites live in mattresses, pillows, and linens such as sheets, blankets, and bedspreads. Even if you have an anti-mite filter or covers for your mattress and your pillow, this will only erase about 5 percent of them, because they also live inside sofas, chairs, upholstered furniture, walls, and carpets.

We suggest you do not keep these types of furniture in your room and that you reduce them to a minimum in the rest of the house. With regard to chairs and sofas, you can choose wooden chairs and leather sofas to keep from accumulating mites. You should also avoid having posters or paintings hung on the walls of your bedroom, and the walls should be painted with washable paint to prevent the accumulation of dust.

What kind of vacuum is the best?

People who are allergic to pollen or mites should always have a vacuum cleaner, because specialists strongly discourage sweeping floors. The best method for

➤

cleaning is to vacuum and mop the floor, and to dust the furniture with a damp cloth or microfiber cloth.

However, not all vacuums can provide satisfactory results in regard to the elimination of mites. Most of them cannot retain particles of less than ten to twenty microns because the bag is porous. Such is the case with mites and their droppings. Therefore we recommend that you use a vacuum with a specific filter called a HEPA (High Efficiency Particulate Air) filter, which prevents the mites from escaping the bag. In addition, it should have strong suction to capture the most dust.

Even more effective than vacuum cleaners or a HEPA filter is a water filter. It works by trapping the mites in water, and they can then be easily disposed of by flushing them down the drain.

What is absolutely not recommended, however, are steam cleaners. The steam, despite its high temperature, creates an optimal environment for dust mites in mattresses, couches, and carpets.

These parasites do not survive in latex or mattresses and pillows because they are made from synthetic materials. However, if you use latex you must first ensure that you do not have an allergic reaction to latex.

If you do not plan to replace your whole mattress, the first major step you can take is to put special anti-mite covers on your mattresses and pillows. These covers are made with an impermeable material that has very small pores that prevent dust mites and their waste from passing to the inside of the mattress. If you prefer to use plastic sheets, this can save some money but is ultimately less comfortable. If your children share a room, you should give the same treatment to their beds, and if they use bunk beds, have the child with the greater sensitivity to mites sleep in the more elevated bed because mites are heavy and do not float in the air. Wash their favorite stuffed animals weekly with hot water and dry on high, or put in the freezer for six hours at a time once a week. This helps reduce the number of mites living in the toy.

Another favorite place for these critters is bedding. Wash the sheets and bedspread every three or four days in hot water, around 140 degrees Farenheit, or wash in warm water and dry with high heat. Although there is no doubt that natural products are preferable to synthetic, when it comes to allergies, people should avoid wool blankets, cotton mattress covers, and down filling. Mites do not live well in synthetic materials and prefer natural fibers.

These are the most important steps you have to take, as the main source of exposure to mites is in bed. It is also recommended that you keep stuffed animals out of your children's rooms, and avoid having rugs or carpets on the floors of your house. Also, use light and synthetic curtains and wash them once a week. If possible, do not let your pets in your bedroom, because even if you're not allergic to their dander, they are a breeding ground for mites and carry their droppings.

When cleaning your house, wear a mask that helps keep you from breathing in allergens, although it is ideal for a member of the household without a dust mite allergy to take responsibility for the cleaning. Clean your house at a time of day when you do not have to go into your bedroom to prevent bringing more mites into that environment.

Avoid having carpets. If you decide to have one, make sure that it is washable and has short, coarse fibers, as they are less hospitable to mites than shaggy carpets. Wash and dry rugs thoroughly at high temperatures, which will help eliminate mites.

As previously mentioned, the mites need a humid environment to thrive, so keep the humidity levels in your house below 50 percent. To achieve this, you can install a dehumidifier or air conditioner. Humidifiers can be helpful in preventing asthma attacks, but harmful when you suffer an allergy to mites. There are many people who feel that the air inside their homes is too dry and that it is healthier to maintain a high humidity level. However, this measure leads to a proliferation of mites and fungi. And, remember, it is the mites that cause your allergy, not dust. In fact, you can live in a house full of dust and have no allergic reactions. You can live in a house full of dust, but if your surrounding environment is very dry and you keep your home well-ventilated you will not have any problems. On the other hand, your home can be very clean but if you are in a wet and warm place, it may be full of mites.

Ventilate your home

Modern homes are well insulated. Windows close perfectly, insulated for the cold and heat, doors fit to keep heat in, but we often forget a basic element that keeps the atmosphere of our home in good condition: ventilation.

We may not have stopped to consider the amount of water vapor that is generated inside our home. And we do not mean only in the kitchen or bathroom, but through our own bodies. Every inhabitant of the house gives off about a quart of moisture daily through perspiration. For example, amounts of moisture in a four-person home can reach twenty-five gallons per week in the form of steam and humidity.

There are two problems to be addressed in the homes of people who suffer from allergies to mites or mold: the high level of humidity in the house, and the areas of condensation that are teeming with mites and fungi.

First, to reduce moisture and humidity, repair cracks in ceilings and walls and check for leaks in the roof or plumbing.

In addition, keep the kitchen and bathroom doors closed while they are in use, and open the windows when you have finished cooking or showering. It is highly recommended to install an exhaust fan in the kitchen or forced ventilation in the bathroom if there are no windows. Do not leave wet towels in the bathroom and dry the walls and the tub to prevent the water from evaporating and increasing the humidity.

It is better to take wet clothes outside or use a dryer, because leaving them indoors helps creates steam.

It is essential to open windows throughout the house for about fifteen minutes every morning, especially if it rains. On very humid days, it is best that you reduce that time by half. If you're looking for a new home, try to pick one that has windows in the front and in the back so you can have cross-ventilation. This will help circulate the air through your home.

➤

75

➤

In an ideal bathroom, there are only tiles in the essential parts like the shower, but the other walls are painted with washable matte paint. Glossy paint, tiles, and plastic develop a lot of condensation on their surfaces. You should not keep carpets in the bathroom, and the windows should have wood or PVC frames, rather than metal, which also holds a lot of moisture. If possible, install a double-glazed window because the inside will be warmer and therefore not condense water vapor.

If you just built your house, the moisture inside is even more elevated as a result of the work and should be ventilated even more, especially during the first year.

And remember, moisture is the best ally of the mites and fungi, which are potent allergens.

Another measure you can use in your fight against mites is anti-mite products. Sold in powder or spray, each has specific forms of application and recommended frequency of use. Normally sofas, carpets, mattresses, and so on should be sprayed every week. Besides anti-mite treatments, fungicides and bactericides can be used for even greater results. However, they may have strong odors that provoke an attack of asthma or rhinitis. Try to choose ones that are made from natural ingredients and whose fragrance is not very strong.

Mold

Molds are a complex group of living organisms found in nature in almost any location, weather, and season. It is impossible to avoid contact with them, and they can be ingested or inhaled. So far eighty thousand species of mold have been identified, but it is believed that that only constitutes 10 percent of total species.

Mold is a fungus and grows both outside and inside the home, near heat and humidity. It is a potent allergen and responsible for many severe cases of asthma. This allergy is very common, and environmental conditions in homes today are conducive to its growth. Unfortunately, there is still a lot more to learn about the nature of these allergens. What has been found is that generally, this allergy also causes a cross-reaction with mites, pollen, or food allergies.

The allergens that trigger the allergic reaction are actually light mold spores that circulate in the air in your home. Many of them are between two and ten microns (one micron is a thousandth of a millimeter) and there are even a few species whose spores are less than 2 microns. This hinders their removal from the environment because they are able to traverse filters and masks without a problem.

Mold grows in all areas where there is moisture, such as on houseplants and in their soil, damp walls, windows, wallpaper, mattresses, beds, basements, attics, pools, greenhouses, and bathrooms. If you live on the ground floor and have moisture in the walls, check to see if the mold is growing from the ground up and is whitish or greenish color: this means the moisture is coming up from the soil.

Butane gas heating and humidifiers complicate the problem more because they increase the humidity in your house and promote areas of condensation where mold grows best.

Mold grows on both natural and synthetic materials, at an ideal temperature of seventy degrees, and a humidity level of 80 percent. People who have asthma triggered by the inhalation of spores have worse symptoms in damp and warm weather, and in autumn when the leaves fallen from trees are decaying. If you are affected in these scenarios then it is almost certain that the source of your allergy is mold.

Each species of mold releases spores differently, although the worst seasons are during the months of February, March, August, and September. Some species release spores at noon, others at night or early morning, and others in the afternoon.

Mold can also grow on fruits, vegetables, grains, yeast, cheese, black pepper, sauerkraut, and nuts, and in alcoholic beverages such as wine, champagne, or beer. If you see mold on an apple, for example, then do not eat it, but there are other species of mold that are microscopic and can be consumed without realizing it. If you find that there are fruits and vegetables that make you feel sick, that discomfort could be caused by a mold allergy instead of a food intolerance.

Furthermore, substances or enzymes from mold are often used in refined products such as leather, soap, detergents, cosmetics, and toothpaste. They can also be used in products that are of biological origin, so look closely at the labels to avoid buying products that can give you allergies.

Penicillin is also a fungus, so if you have a serious allergy to fungus, you may also have a reaction to this drug.

Alternaria

Spores from fungus are responsible for many cases of asthma. Alternaria is one of the most common fungi that grow outdoors. It lives in fallen leaves, plants, and decaying organic material, but the spores float in the air. It is found in houses in window frames, where condensation of atmospheric moisture occurs.

Spores are released all year, especially on hot and humid days. They enter homes through the windows, but the ratio of indoor to outdoor air is approximately four to one.

It causes allergic rhinoconjunctivitis and bronchial asthma, and it can produce pneumonitis in individuals hypersensitive to this allergen. It is very powerful and can cause fatal outcomes in patients with allergies. In fact, it is one of the major causes of childhood asthma and asthma in people living with continuing exposure to Alternaria in damp places with organic material (lawns, gardens, or orchards).

Symptoms of an allergy to this fungus are more common in late spring and autumn.

How to remove mold from your home. The symptoms of an allergic person are greatly improved if the level of humidity is decreased. So, as we've discussed in the section on "ventilate your home," the only solution to rid your house of mold is mainly to prevent condensation and maintain areas of the house with a low degree of humidity. It is a good idea to air out your house or install air conditioning with a heat pump (hot and cold air). It can also help to have a dehumidifier that you can put in the rooms that are a particular source of moisture. It is essential to fix any leaks and clear up dampness in the walls.

In addition, there are other solutions to combat moisture from the walls on the ground floors. A professional injects a special liquid into the walls that seals the pores of the brick and prevents soil moisture from "climbing" up. The injections are made every few feet and within months the walls are dry and the mold disappears. Another method to dry the walls is to install wall electrodes that draw moisture back to the ground instead of allowing it to climb up. These electrodes are connected to a central unit that operates at very low power (like a battery) and keeps your walls dry. Both methods are expensive and require some work, but are guaranteed to solve the problem.

Furthermore, there are products on the market that kill mold. You should read the labels carefully because these products contain strong chemicals that can provoke other reactions, and you should clean the dead mold that remains because that can produce an allergic reaction as well. Other products that are great for cleaning mold are the alcohol you have in your medicine cabinet, and bleach, but you should not mix them. Places where mold generally grows are metal window frames, bathrooms, kitchens, rubber edges of the door of the refrigerator and freezer, or air conditioners, among other places, not to mention the basement and walls, and objects that contain moisture. However, if the problem is still not resolved after thoroughly cleaning the mold, spores will return and settle in your home once again.

Also, do not keep indoor plants at home because their leaves and soil usually proliferate mold. In addition, you should carefully wash fruits and vegetables and, if possible, always peel fruit before you eat it.

You should not buy industrial products that may contain mold enzymes. Buy toothpaste powder instead of paste, and use soap flakes or neutral soap instead of detergent. It is difficult to distinguish which products are enzymes of mold in their composition because the manufacturer is not required to identify it on the label, so you should check with them directly. However, it is best to choose the safest option, and using a natural soap will help you avoid unnecessary risks.

You should get rid of all furniture that has a musty smell, because that smell means it is infested with mold. Moreover, clothes and curtains that contain mold should be washed thoroughly or replaced.

And remember that while it is difficult to eradicate mold entirely, you can control the temperature, humidity, and condensation-prone areas, helping you to better cope with day-to-day life in your home.

Animals

Coming into contact with a dog, cat, rabbit, hamster, horse, or even a bird can cause pet allergies. Actually, what produces the allergic reaction is not the hair of the animal itself, as is commonly believed. The allergen is usually found in small flakes of dead skin that the animal releases, in their saliva, and even in their urine, as in the case of rabbits, guinea pigs, and hamsters. The allergen comes in contact with your skin or is inhaled.

Cat allergens are the smallest and also the most powerful. They are very small and very slight saliva particles floating in the air or are left in its hair when the cat fails to maintain daily hygiene. Many of these particles are smaller than two and a half microns and smaller ones measure up to a half micron. In the case of dogs, there are also allergens in particles of their saliva, but they are less potent. Also, because dogs do not wash with their own saliva as cats do, these allergens do not spread as much.

The data does not lie. Cat or dog allergies occur in about 15 percent of the population. For those with asthma, the percentage rises to 20 or 30 percent. If it is contact dermatitis, this allergy can cause itching and hives. Symptoms usually occur within minutes of exposure to an animal. For some people with late-phase allergies, symptoms can develop over several hours and become serious as long as twelve hours after discontinuing contact with the animal.

The best solution in the case of an allergy to pets is to give the animal up for adoption and eliminate any trace of it at home. However, you will still encounter dog or cat allergens in many other places such as in public places or on public transportation, as the owners of pets can transport these allergens on their clothes. In cases of hypersensitivity to the saliva of these animals, people can have a difficult time finding relief from their symptoms.

However, if you decide to keep your pet, it will be very difficult to overcome the symptoms because it is almost impossible to remove their allergens. You can greatly reduce their presence, but this is only half a solution.

There are allergic people who resist getting rid of their cat or dog because they argue that there is no direct reaction, that their symptoms are not as bad if they brush their pet, or if they keep them out of their bedrooms. This does not mean that the allergy does not exist, but it is hidden. This usually occurs when a person is in constant daily contact with their allergen. For example, someone with an allergy to wheat who eats bread every day may not feel bad right after consuming it, but will eventually have an attack anyway. In the case of allergies to animals, it is the same. If the allergy test result shows reactivity to the protein from the saliva of your pet, there is no doubt that you have an allergy, although there is no direct reaction.

However, we must also say that there are other medical theories that argue that the coexistence of pets and newborns helps keep children from developing allergies later, and that excessively sterile environments do not allow the child's immune system to mature. However, this effect does not occur if the parents smoke at home because, as we will see, cigarette smoke is one of the greatest causes of respiratory allergies.

Who will take care of my pet?

Often, when a person who is allergic to animals decides to get rid of their pet in order to completely eradicate his ailment, there are many questions about how to do this.

It is difficult to find a new satisfactory home for our much-loved pet. Generally, people prefer to buy or adopt a puppy and it seems an impossible task to find your older pet a new home.

However, do not despair, because there are different ways to find a new place for them to live. For example, you can try to put ads in local publications or specialized Internet portals on pet adoption. There are also associations that are responsible for resolving adoptions, and you can also relate your problem to your family, friends, and neighbors in the hopes that they or someone they know can provide a good home. Sometimes, people are more likely to adopt an animal when the issue is as serious your health.

Furthermore, nursing homes and elderly people prefer adult dogs and quiet and well-behaved cats to keep them company, rather than face the arduous task of teaching habits and manners to a naughty puppy.

Remedies for animal allergies. The ideal solution with full guarantees is to not have animals at home. It's that drastic.

However, there is evidence that this measure, which is the most effective, is not taken by most people. So we will provide a number of strategies that, while they will not solve the problem entirely, may provide some improvement in your symptoms. They are somewhat difficult to follow because you have to be constantly on top of these tasks, but sometimes it is still more difficult to give up an old dog that you love, so you must weigh the situation and be sure of the decision you make.

First of all, it is imperative that you keep your pet out of your bedroom entirely. Who does not like to sleep with their cat or have their dog at the foot of the bed? But if you are allergic to their saliva, this pleasant companionship has come to an end, at least when it comes to your room.

This measure should also apply to the rest of the house, especially in places where you spend the most time, like the dining room, study, kitchen, or bathroom. However, your shoes and your clothes can transport their potent allergens from one place to another, thus it is difficult to find relief in your home even in rooms where your pet is not allowed.

So ideally, if you have a deck or patio, your cat or dog should spend most of their time outdoors. Make sure their space is comfortable. If other people living with you want to play with the pet, remind them that they should change clothes and shoes afterwards to avoid tracking the allergens into the house.

Bathing your pet weekly reduces the amount of allergens released, but bi-weekly is ideal as your pet re-releases these allergens every three days. Consult your veterinarian about what shampoos are safe to use. Have a member of your household who does not have a pet allergy bathe the pet, as it may cause you to have a strong reaction.

The same goes for brushing your pet. Brushing your pet daily outside of the house is quite effective for reducing dander, but it is best to have someone who is not affected by the allergens take care of it. Clean their crate or cage weekly, as well.

Cats and dogs produce allergens continuously, although the amount produced varies greatly from pet to pet. Allergens build up in rugs, mattresses, pillows, and even walls and floors. They can penetrate fibers, so you should use allergenic pillowcases and furniture covers to keep particles from settling inside the cushions.

Vacuuming does not entirely solve the problem, as it does not clean carpets very thoroughly, and in fact, often stirs up particles during cleaning. A HEPA filter is helpful for trapping these particles and keeping them from re-entering your environment.

Installing an air-purifier with a HEPA filter will help capture particles in the air. Allergens are very light and float through the air, and a filter can both catch them in large quantities and trap them successfully. Purifiers cannot protect you from the dander your cat sheds on surfaces, however, though some manufacturers advertise as such.

Avoid sprays that advertise that they "kill" allergens when sprayed on your cat or dog, because studies have proven that these do not work.

Insect Bites and Stings

Typically, a sting from a bee, wasp, or other insect produces a reaction with pain, itching, swelling, and redness that disappears within a few days. But if the bite affects an allergic person, the reaction is much stronger and can send the person into anaphylactic shock.

Bites that cause an allergic reaction usually come from the family of Hymenoptera insects, which is comprised of three species: wasps, bees, and ants.

Did you know...

Allergic reactions to insect bites and stings have been documented since the beginning of the human race. One of the first records of this was found in ancient Egypt, where hieroglyphics from the Tomb of Pharoah Menes show his death by a wasp sting. Even after thousands of years, allergic reactions caused by the bites of wasps, bees, and certain ants remain a serious medical problem that requires urgent treatment.

COMMON ALLERGENS: HOW TO COMBAT THEIR EFFECTS

Though severe allergic reactions to insect bites are not very common, when they do occur, the reaction can affect many organs and develop extremely quickly, resulting in anaphylactic shock. Symptoms may include hives over large areas of the body, swelling in the throat or tongue, difficulty breathing, dizziness, abdominal discomfort, nausea, or diarrhea. In extreme cases, it causes a rapid drop in blood pressure that can put the body into shock and cause the patient to lose consciousness. These symptoms require emergency medical treatment as this reaction can be fatal.

To avoid being stung or bitten by these insects it is essential that you learn to recognize them by following the wisdom of "know your enemy." Insects that commonly cause allergic reactions are yellow jackets, honeybees, wasps, and hornets.

"Yellow jackets" have characteristic black-and-yellow markings and are found in different climates. Their nests, which are made of a material similar to cellulose, are usually built underground, but are also on the walls of buildings, in cracks in walls, or in woodpiles.

Honeybees have a rounded and hairy dark brown body with yellow markings. The honeybee is not aggressive and only stings when it is provoked or feels threatened. Domesticated honeybees are kept in hives, but wild honeybees build their hives in hollow trees or cavities of buildings.

Unlike bees, wasps have slender, elongated bodies, and they can be black, brown, or red, with yellow stripes. They make their nests with paper-like material forming circular cells that make a honeycomb shape. They are built under the eaves in roofs, behind shutters, or in shrubs or woodpiles.

Hornets are black, orange, yellow, or brown, with white markings, and they are larger than yellow jackets. Their nests are gray or brown, with melon-shaped cells similar to the cellulose nests of yellow jackets.

They tend to live in the branches of trees, shrubs, or in hollow trees. They are mostly active between May and September, and especially in July and August, as the summer heat causes the wasps to become even more active.

Honeybees are attracted to the fragrance of flowers, bright colors, and smooth wet surfaces. Wasps feed on sugary liquids such as juices, sap, and nectar. However, some wasps feed on other insects when the wasps are in the larval stage. This is why wasps use venom: to paralyze future food sources for their larvae. Unlike bees, wasps do not lose their stingers and can sting multiple times. This does not occur in bees, as their stingers have a serrated tracer that becomes anchored in the tissue of their victim and tears loose part of the bee's abdomen; and so bees can only sting once, and then they die.

If you are stung by an insect but did not see what kind of insect stung you, look for their stinger in your skin. You should remove it carefully to avoid pressing on the venom sac and inadvertently emptying its entire contents. Remove the stinger as soon as possible, as the venom gland from the bee is attached to the stinger, and will continue to periodically release venom into your skin until it is emptied.

If you do not find a stinger, it is likely that you were stung by a wasp. In that case you should know that when a wasp stings, it releases a pheromone that attracts other members of the colony, and you need to leave the location in which you were stung immediately to avoid being attacked by more wasps.

Cross-reactions between wasps, hornets, and other insects in the vespid family are common, so if you are allergic to one kind of sting, you will also have similar reactions to other kinds. However, it is rare to suffer cross-reactions between bee and wasp reactions.

Honeybees and bumblebees have very similar venom, and it is common to have a cross-reaction to both. There is also a cross-reaction between bumblebee venom and snake venom. People are also commonly allergic to ant bites, and these bites can also cause anaphylaxis. Cross-reactions between wasps and ants are common as well. These ants are reddish brown and live in protruding mounds up to 90 cm in diameter and 45 cm high. These nests may contain up to 250,000 ants, so you should avoid approaching, hitting, or disturbing a nest if you find one. Red ants can also strike without warning and in a very unpleasant way: they firmly grab their victim's skin with their mandibles, arch their back, and insert their stinger into the skin. Then they pivot around the stinger about eight times in a circle. Their sting is quite painful.

How to prevent insect bites. There are several precautions you can take to avoid being stung by a bee or a wasp. They are not an absolute guarantee, but may help you on more than one occasion.

As is logical, you should not approach a honeycomb or a wasp's nest. But if you happen to make contact with a bee or wasp, try not to kill or scare it. The insect will interpret this as an attack and act in self-defense by attacking with its stinger. Instead, try to remain motionless or make slow movements while you walk away.

When you leave clothes on the floor or outside shops, shake them out before you wear them because they could be hiding a wasp or a bee in one of their folds.

If you go outside, wear long sleeves, and avoid bright colors and perfumes to keep from attracting insects. Also, it is best to avoid walking through areas dense with flowers, as they attract a huge number of insects.

It is advisable not to keep the car windows open when you travel in the summer, not only to avoid being stung, but also to avoid being the victim of an accident by trying to get the insect out of the vehicle. If a bee or wasp stings you while you're traveling in a fast-moving vehicle, this can cause a serious bite as the impact makes the insect release all of its venom at once. This can also happen when you're traveling by motorcycle and do not wear enough protective clothing. When on a bicycle or on horseback, the bite will not be as powerful, as you are a moving at a slower rate, but if you have an allergy to insect bites, it is best to not risk exposure.

If you drink sweet drinks outdoors in the summer, pay special attention when raising your glass to your mouth, as it is likely that a greedy wasp or bee is on the edge of your glass.

Make sure you have screens in your windows and use suitable insecticides at night. Always supervise children to make sure they do not throw objects at insect nests.

Avoid red ants and anthills. Do not touch their nests under any circumstances. We tend to believe that ants are harmless, but this is not the case.

How to treat a sting. If you suffer from allergies these insects bites will provoke local inflammation. In that case, apply ointment and cold compresses to soothe itching and pain. If the bite is very painful, you can use an oral antihistamine or anti-inflammatory as a last resort to relieve discomfort. The bite will heal in a few days.

Make a paste with hot water and tablets of activated charcoal, and apply it to the affected area with a piece of gauze or clean, damp cotton. These tablets are sold in health stores, and you should always carry some when you go for a walk outdoors.

If you are allergic to Hymenoptera stings, these will cause a more severe reaction. Symptoms include fever, and swelling of joints or limbs, among others. If this happens, you should see a doctor and take an allergy test to learn what insect exactly caused this reaction and how sensitive you are to their sting.

As we've mentioned before, these insect stings can cause anaphylactic shock in some patients. In these cases the patient should seek medical advice immediately and carry an EpiPen and an antihistamine to keep the reaction under control.

Latex

Latex is a substance that is obtained from the sap of the *Hevea brasiliensis* tree, also known as "the rubber tree."

Modern life has brought a great demand for this product, and latex can be found in many everyday products, such as gloves, balloons, toys, synthetic nipples and pacifiers, preservatives, diaphragms, shoe soles, sports equipment, and dental material. Also, the latex has found a wide range of applications in the world of medicine in surgical materials such as gloves, probes, catheters, masks, elastic bandages, etc.

A latex allergy affects 1 percent of the population of industrialized countries where latex is everywhere.

Most problematically, latex is found everywhere in medical and hospital environments. This means that when a person with a latex allergy goes to the doctor they are exposed to contact with latex objects and can suffer an allergic reaction. Therefore it is essential to wear clear identification in a visible place stating that you are allergic to latex.

Latex can produce two types of allergic reactions: immediate or delayed. The first produces contact dermatitis and the second produces symptoms such as hives, asthma, conjunctivitis, rhinitis, and anaphylaxis. It is more common in children.

The patient should avoid all contact, direct or indirect, with items containing latex. Also, do not forget that the latex particles can remain suspended in the air for hours, especially in operating rooms after the use of gloves.

Cross-reactions with latex and certain fruits are common. This can be explained because they contain the same enzyme, called "chitinase," which protects plants from insect pests.

Type of cross reaction	Food
Common and important	Banana, avocado, kiwi, chestnut
Important but rare	Potato, seafood
Frequently according to statistics	Papaya, tomato, pineapple, mango, fig, nuts, melon, cherry, apple
Infrequent	Guava, fish, carrot, pear, strawberry, peanut, pepper, grape
Isolated cases	Cocoa, oregano, sage, milk, spinach, green beans, beets

Foods

There are many potential allergens and cross-reactions found in food. Some reactions occur just as soon as the food enters the mouth, so that food allergens are easily identified and can be eliminated from your diet. However, when a late reaction occurs, it is more difficult to detect the cause. In those cases, a food allergy can manifest itself in digestive problems, a cough, or an irritating tickle in the throat, but food can cause other symptoms such as rhinitis or asthma, which do not necessarily point to the ingestion of food as a source.

In food allergies, sometimes the perpetrators are proteins that are found in food, and other times, reactions are caused by chemical additives that are added to processed or refined food. This could explain how the presence of food allergies in people has increased in recent decades. A study showed that in France between 1984 and 1992, severe food allergies had been caused mainly by allergens from processed foods.

In principle, any food can cause an allergic reaction, and medical literature has documented about 170 foods that cause allergic reactions. Among them, several are the most common. These are called the "big eight" and include: milk, eggs, peanuts, tree nuts, fish, shellfish, soy, and wheat. This group is the cause of 90 percent of all food allergies. The remaining 10 percent include eight others, the "second eight": sesame and other seeds—sunflower, cotton and poppy—beans, peas, lentils, tartrazine, sulfites, and latex.

However, allergies can be caused by any other food that is not referenced in this group of sixteen. This broad spectrum makes it difficult to establish a diagnosis of allergies to food products, because in many cases the symptoms are not well defined. In addition, interactions between the hormonal system and the nervous system are also a factor, and produce very subtle symptoms. For example, a scientific study has shown that people with food allergies can develop a reaction without having any direct contact with the allergen. This is due to the neurotransmitter acetylcholine and explains why people who are allergic to fish sometimes get an itchy mouth just from looking at fish in the store.

Furthermore, there is a high incidence of cross-reactive factors. If you are allergic to one food, you will also be allergic to foods within the same family. For example, if you are allergic to onions, you will also react to garlic because both foods belong to the Liliaceae family.

Symptoms of food allergies are not limited to gastrointestinal problems or issues with the absorption of nutrients. An allergy to the protein in cow's milk can produce asthma or rhinitis, or even hives. Symptoms can be quite varied and differ in intensity. It may provoke a slightly itchy mouth that disappears after a while or anaphylactic shock requiring hospital admission. If you do not act quickly in this case, consequences can be fatal. Most anaphylactic reactions occur in patients who know they have an allergy to a certain food, but are unaware that what they have just eaten contains this ingredient, either due to lack of knowledge, a careless mistake, or because it is not specified on the product label.

Sometimes an allergy can also be caused by cross-reactions, such as between onions and garlic, or celery and carrots.

Although over time one can develop a certain tolerance to foods that originally caused an allergy, such as milk or eggs, there are cases where the sensitivity will continue for the rest of the patient's life, especially in the case of fish, shellfish, peanuts, and dried fruits. In these cases, doctors recommend completely eliminating the allergenic food from the patient's diet.

In addition to allergy testing you can use a personal diagnosis for potential allergens. First, if you've noticed any immediate reaction from eating a certain food, do not consume that food for a week, and then reintroduce it to your diet and check for a reaction. Never eat that particular food in large quantities. Only consume it in small quantities accompanied by other foods to minimize the reaction and avoid anaphylactic shock. However, it is not always this simple, as the reaction can manifest immediately or may only occur because of the combination of several foods at once.

Below we will describe some of the most allergenic foods.

Cow's milk. Man is the only mammal that drinks milk for their whole lives, processing the milk of other species to do so, especially cows in industrialized countries. Once children are weaned off of their mother's milk, their levels of enzymes that help digest the lactose in cow's milk decrease, causing lactose intolerance later in their life.

Each species of mammal produces its own specific milk to feed their offspring. Although cow's milk may look like human milk, it is not. The fat content and size of the proteins of cow's milk are much greater than what is ideal for human metabolism. In addition, the proportions of carbohydrates and minerals are also different.

Also, milk provides the baby (or calf) with hormones, antibodies, and other species-specific immunological elements.

In addition to causing an increase in secretion of mucous and providing high levels of fat, milk contains two nutrients that often cause problems for the human metabolism: lactose and casein.

Lactose is the sugar in milk. Our body produces an enzyme called "lactase," which helps to properly digest lactose. However, people's lactase levels decrease as a person becomes an adult, because our metabolism was only prepared to digest milk as infants. This deficit does not allow lactase to digest lactose sugar and this can cause us to develop an intolerance. This phenomenon can occur both in adults and also in infants. The symptoms associated with lactose intolerance are diarrhea, malnutrition, abdominal distension, bloating, abdominal cramps, and weight loss. There are also other associated symptoms such as joint problems or muscle pain that make it less clear that the origin of these symptoms is lactose intolerance.

Casein is one of 25 milk proteins and is found in the milk of every species, including humans. However, the size of this protein is not the same in all species. A baby can fully assimilate caseins of milk from her mother, but cannot do the same with caseins from cow's milk, which are much larger and pass into the small intestine without being digested at all because it also neutralizes the stomach acid required to break down these proteins. This problem is exacerbated in adults because the amount of gastric rennin decreases with age. Rennin is the first enzyme required to launch the chain reaction that breaks down large molecules of casein. Our metabolism is designed to best digest milk in only the first years of life.

People who are allergic to casein should note that this protein is present in all dairy (milk, cheese, yogurt), and most problematically, processed cheese that contains a higher concentration. If you like cheese, eat cheeses that are naturally prepared from milk through fermentation methods for a lesser allergic reaction to the casein.

Milk, a highly refined product

Cow's milk has been modified over time. The white liquid with which we fill our glass today has little to do with what they served to our grandparents. Nowadays, industrial processes have modified the milk to allow for a longer shelf life. Unprocessed milk is not readily available, except in more remote areas.

There are several processes that the food industry applies to cow's milk. First, they use methods of sterilization such as pasteurization, UHT, etc. In these processes, the milk is heated to high temperatures and then rapidly cooled. The goal of this heating and cooling is to eliminate germs, but it does not remove the milk hormones and antibiotics that are fed to cows to increase milk production. This makes the milk less perishable and able to be stored for many months, but the nutritive properties are altered after being subjected to heat. Then chemical additives are incorporated to further modify the milk.

Homogenization is another manufacturing process that is used to improve the texture of milk. It reduces the size of fat globules by at least ten times.

There is a great effort from the food industry to manage problems associated with their products. If doctors say that whole milk is bad for cholesterol, they invent skimmed milk. If skimmed milk has too watery a texture, they come up with part-skim; if the milk has lost fat soluble vitamins, they add vitamins A and D; calcium is added to help reduce the risk of osteoporosis; Omega-3 fatty acids are added to reduce cholesterol; low lactose milk is manufactured for people who have a hard time digesting milk; if the consumer wants more fiber, they add more fiber; they create "enriched" milk for children, milk with twelve vitamins and minerals...You see, natural milk is only a vague memory, and your body is faced with a highly refined product full of synthetic additives.

People with a casein allergy have to take into account that it is not only present in milk.

Due to the high demand of low-fat products, the dairy industry adds it to many substances, including cream.

There are people who only drink small amounts of milk, if any at all, but suffer a reaction to casein. It is important to read product labels and make sure that the products they consume do not contain dairy additives. For example, the vast majority of processed baked goods such as bread, cookies, or pastries contain some dairy additive such as cream, milk solids, whey, milk proteins, or milk powder.

How can I substitute dairy in my diet?

Milk
There are many healthy and nutritious alternatives to dairy milk, called "plant-based milks." The most common is made from soybeans, but other milk alternatives are made from oats, rice, almonds, hazelnuts, and horchata. You can make these at home, or buy them in bottles and cartons.

Soy can be used in the preparation of many different foods such as sauces, creams, cakes, or desserts.

Butter
Most margarine found in the grocery store incorporates some dairy, such as serum or skim milk. You need to look for completely plant-based margarines. If you are using margarine made from palm or coconut oil, use them in moderation because even though they are plant-based, they contain high amounts of saturated fats.

Dairy Desserts
Yogurt and custard can also be prepared from soy milk. You can buy them in the store, or make them at home with cultures sold in health food stores. The benefits of live cultures in yogurt do not depend on the kind of milk used to make it, so you can keep probiotics in your diet.

Cheese
Cheeses that come from non-dairy milks like soy are produced using the same process used to make cheese from animal milk. Soy milk cheese—tofu—has the texture of cheese and can be used in a numerous dishes. In the case of cured cheeses, results are not as similar to dairy.

> **Ice Cream**
>
> Ice cream is made from cream, and very few establishments have non-dairy options. However, on a hot day, some refreshing options include horchata, slushies, and fruit sorbets. If you have a freezer at home, you can always make your own ice cream from soy milk and use whatever flavors you like.

Eggs. Eggs are a very complete and rich food high in valuable proteins and B vitamins They also supply lipids necessary for the formation of cell membranes and various organic substances such as hormones.

Both the white and the yolk contain many proteins, so both can cause allergic reactions, especially in children. The reaction can generate high levels of IgE, triggered by twenty-four different glycoproteins. The proteins that cause the strongest reactions are ovotransferrin, ovalbumin, and ovomucoid. The yolk is introduced earlier in the diet of children because it is less allergenic, but can also cause allergic reaction through the livetins. This substance is present in chicken feathers, meat, and eggs, which explains the appearance of the bird-egg syndrome, which causes allergic reactions from the inhalation of particles of feathers or other substances present in birds. Cross-reactions occur between the proteins in the yolk and the white of the egg, as well as between different kinds of birds and their eggs.

When a child is born, their diet is limited to breast milk or infant formula. As the baby grows, the mother begins incorporating different foods as the pediatrician advises. Egg allergies do not develop until you have incorporated the yolk into your diet. It is an allergy that is usually outgrown over the years, which does not happen for other allergenic foods such as nuts, legumes, fish, or shellfish, which produce allergies that last for a lifetime.

If a child is allergic to eggs, they should be removed completely from their diet. Eggs do not contain any essential nutrients that cannot be supplied through other foods, but they are found in a large range of processed foods to help with stabilization and emulsification among other things. Manufacturers are not required to include the egg ingredient on their labels.

Eggs can be found in the following:

- Soups, broths, or consommés clarified with egg.
- Breaded meat, deli meat, burgers, cakes, pies.
- Bakery products, bread, rolls, cakes, cookies, puddings, custards, meringues.
- Sauces containing egg, like mayonnaise or tartar sauce.
- Ice cream and sorbets.
- Mixed-milk products such as eggnog and smoothies.
- Beverages such as coffee or wine with clarified egg white, extracts containing egg whites as a foaming agent.
- Other sources include egg macaroni, noodles, nougat, caramels, and many frozen foods.

As you can see, the list is extensive. Thus, you should read the labels of food products and reject those containing whole, powdered, or dehydrated eggs, as well as albumin, globulin, livetin, lecithin, soybeans, lysozyme, ovalbumin, ovomucin, ovomucoid, ovovitelina, or E161B (lutein, a yellow pigment).

Vaccines

The administration of vaccines prepared in embryonated chicken or duck egg, such as those for the flu, yellow fever, or rabies, can produce an allergic reaction. While there are arguments for and against the administration of vaccines, it is necessary to get the vaccination in a hospital setting where they can control a hypothetical anaphylactic shock.

In contrast, vaccines prepared in human diploid cells, such as those for measles, rubella, or mumps, do not contain yolk components or ovalbumin (egg allergenic substances), so you can have them administered safely.

Different studies claim that complications can occur with the following vaccines:

- Anti-flu
- Yellow fever
- Measles
- Mumps
- MMR (measles-mumps-rubella)

Vaccines that do not present any risk to people allergic to eggs include:

- DPT (diphtheria, tetanus, pertussis)
- Rubella
- Tetanus

Fish. Saltwater fish is the source of a large percentage of food allergies. This is a common allergy caused by proteins the fish contain called "parvalbumins." These proteins are very similar in all saltwater fish, so if you are allergic to hake, it is very likely that you are also allergic to cod and sardines.

As you know, fish is a food that should be consumed shortly after being captured because it is a very perishable product. Within hours, the tissue begins to decompose and this process generates a high content of histamine. It can also cause allergic reactions in people who are sensitive to this substance or who have high levels of histamine in their body.

In addition to its protein and histamine content, it was recently found that there is a third cause of allergy found in fish. This is the parasite Anisakis simplex that can grow a few inches long. When in the larval stage, it lives in the digestive tract of many fish like hake, tuna, cod, cephalopods (cuttlefish, octopus, and squid), and crustaceans (lobsters, crayfish, crabs). This parasite can enter our stomach if we eat undercooked, raw, pickled, salted, smoked, or marinated fish.

There are two types of disease caused by this parasite: intolerance or allergy. The first is when the parasite reaches the gastrointestinal mucosa and causes digestive problems. The second is an allergic reaction due to the intervention of IgE. In these cases it can be severe because it can lead to anaphylactic shock. There are documented cases of cross-reactions with other nematodes, arthropods, mites, cockroaches, and shrimp.

If you find that you are allergic to fish protein you should also keep in mind that you may be allergic to meat from animals that have been fed with fishmeal, as is the case with pork or chicken. The most common symptoms are: rash, cutaneous itching, and difficulty breathing. Children with asthma or atopic dermatitis often get worse if they eat fish.

Unfortunately, allergies caused by fish can accompany you throughout life. If so, the only truly effective solution is to not eat any type of fish or any food that may contain fish-derived components.

Seafood. Allergens in seafood are found in the muscular system and the skin. This is the tropomyosin protein essential in muscle contraction in both invertebrates and vertebrates. Thus, cases were recorded involving cross-reactions with insects, mites, nematodes, and various kinds of mollusks, because they contain the same protein. So chances are if you are allergic to dust mites, you may also have more or less intense reactions when consuming seafood, shellfish, or crustaceans.

It should be noted, moreover, that while fish allergies constitute 18 percent of all cases of food allergy in children (almost one in five cases), reactions to crustaceans and mollusks constitute 3.8 percent and 1.6 percent respectively.

Nuts. Nut allergies are very common, and typically triggered by walnuts, almonds, hazelnuts, and peanuts (which are legumes like lentils and peas). The allergens produced by the proteins present in nuts and seeds are the same as the proteins found in certain pollens. Therefore, if you have been diagnosed with hay fever, you may have a cross-reaction with some kinds of nuts.

The allergens found in the seed of the nut can be destroyed through roasting, but they may be resistant to heat and produce new allergens.

Allergies to nuts can begin at an early age and last your entire lifetime. This allergy can be fatal. It can cause symptoms through ingestion, skin contact, or inhalation, even in small quantities.

Symptoms of a mild allergy can be limited to rash, nausea, headaches, and swelling of the tongue and lips, but a more serious allergy can cause anaphylactic shock.

As with other food allergies, it is best to completely eliminate nuts and nut-based products such as peanut butter or nut-based oils from your diet. There are many products on the market that may contain traces of peanuts or nuts, such as chocolate, cream, cocoa, or chocolate pastries. It is essential that you read the labels of products before purchasing them to avoid having a severe allergic reaction.

Wheat and grains. The major allergens in wheat and grains are proteins such as lecithin that protect the grain from attack by fungi, bacteria, or insects. Thus, the type of allergy differs from person to person, depending on the amount of wheat and grains in their diet.

People who consume a Mediterranean diet are more likely to develop an allergy to wheat, while Northern Europeans are more likely to develop an allergy to rye, or in the case of Asians, rice. In the event that you develop a wheat allergy, your diet will have to be extremely modified because it is used in a wide range of processed foods, including some you would never consider. For this reason, once you are diagnosed with a wheat allergy, it is essential that you read all food labels to make sure you are buying wheat-free food. This is not always clear, so below you will find a list of wheat-derived ingredients:

- Bread crumbs.
- Wheat-bran.
- Malt.
- Couscous.
- Crackers.
- Enriched flour.
- Whole wheat flour.
- Unsifted wheat flour.
- Flour with a high gluten content.
- Flour with a high protein content.
- Wheat-germ.
- Wheat-starch.
- Gelatinized starch.
- Hydrolyzed vegetable protein.
- Modified food starch.
- Soy sauce.
- Starch.
- Rubber plant.
- Vegetable starch.

Furthermore, the gluten from wheat and other grains is responsible for the disease known as "gluten intolerance" or "celiac disease." Although these cases are not IgE-mediated allergies, the symptoms are important to note, and these diseases impact our body's ability to absorb nutrients.

The main problems occur in the intestine, whose protective mucous becomes damaged and inflamed. The discomforts that accompany this intolerance are nausea, vomiting, diarrhea, malnutrition, fatigue, irritability, and abdominal pain.

Food Additives. Although the origin of most food allergies are the proteins found in foods, there is also a low incidence of reactions that are caused by some of the many chemical additives that the food industry incorporates into processed foods to improve their color, flavor, or to make them less perishable.

These substances help food manufacturers to earn more from their products, but they often cause food intolerances and even allergies.

Some are natural and others synthetic, that is, they are created in laboratories. The food industry has been using them for many years, and there are very few packaged foods that do not contain them. There are some products, such as candy, which consist only of chemical additives and sugar.

As consumers, we have been exposed to such a wide range of additives that our digestive systems have been modified, causing the development of food intolerances and adverse reactions to these additives.

Among chemical additives, the most commonly used dyes are tartrazine (E102), quinoline yellow (E104), sunset yellow (E110), azorubine (E122), cochineal red A (E124), the Allura red (E129), and patent blue (E131). They are used in most candies, causing increased cases of food allergies and intolerances in children.

Tartrazine (E102) may cause side effects, although not severe, in asthmatic people and 10 percent of people allergic to aspirin. Symptoms range from nervousness to more adverse reactions, such as hives or breathing problems.

There are also other additives that cause reactions, such as aspartame, benzoates, monosodium glutamate (found in

Chinese food and many sauces), nitrates and nitrites, parabens, and sulfites.

Chemical Products

Some beauty products, clothing detergents, solvents, or other chemicals cause symptoms like hives in sensitive individuals. These substances are formed by proteins that make up common allergens and irritants that produce identical symptoms to intolerances and allergies. These products include dyes, cosmetics, cleaning products for household and industrial use, solvents, paints, and pesticides to treat plants. But there are countless chemicals in our environments that could cause an allergic reaction.

Chemicals are everywhere in our daily lives, such as in synthetic drugs that treat illnesses and pesticides and treatments used in agriculture. Furthermore, despite efforts to consume products of biological origin, and use natural soaps and in our activities, we are surrounded by painted furniture, plastic paints, and synthetic materials.

These chemicals can enter our bodies in different ways: inhalation when they are in the form of steam, such as formaldehyde, varnish, furniture cleaners, certain perfumes, or cosmetics; through the skin, such as creams, or direct contact with paints or solvents; through ingestion, as in the case of pesticides used in agriculture; and contact with eyes, such as with vapors or spray detergents. Whatever way they enter our bodies, these chemicals can get into the bloodstream, where they are distributed throughout our bodies, causing damage both at the entry point, and in other organs they end up reaching.

Allergies to chemicals could be the cause of certain diseases of unknown origin and autoimmune character, such as fibromyalgia, chronic fatigue syndrome, cancer, Alzheimer's, Parkinson's, and even autism. Although this theory generates controversy in the scientific world, it is supported by research.

When many symptoms occur, this can be called "multiple chemical sensitivity syndrome." This disease, which is usually combined with fibromyalgia or chronic fatigue syndrome, causes problems ranging from a minor discomfort to a total disability. The most common symptoms are depression, pruritus, skin blemishes, fainting, dizziness, confusion, memory loss, difficulty breathing, headache, chest pain, muscle pain, fatigue, inability to concentrate, eye, nose, and throat irritation, malaise, indisposition, uneasiness, and gastrointestinal problems.

The worst thing about this condition is that, once triggered, it only takes the slightest traces of exposure to the toxic agent to cause symptoms in the patient.

Medications

When it comes to drug allergies, each and every drug that exists today can cause allergies. However, there are very few people with drug allergies, and these allergies are most commonly linked to aspirin, penicillin, sulfa, barbiturates, anticonvulsants, insulin preparations (including animal-based insulin), local anesthetics such as Novocain, and iodine (found in contrast media for X-rays).

These allergies can cause symptoms including hives, vomiting, diarrhea, respiratory distress, rhinoconjunctivitis, or anaphylaxis.

Hives can break out after the first time you take a medication, causing itching and swelling, especially in the face. Taking the drug again, or taking another drug in the same pharmacological family, will likely increase the severity of the reaction.

The probability that a drug will cause an allergic reaction depends on its chemical makeup and structure. Drugs that most commonly cause allergic reactions include antibiotics, anti-inflammatories, cough syrups, and local anesthetics.

Some drug reactions are rare side effects of the drug in question, such as non-allergic urticaria (without antibodies), aspirin, or an asthma attack.

People sometimes confuse uncomfortable, but not serious, side effects of a medication, such as nausea, with allergy symptoms. Allergies to drugs only include those reactions mediated by the immune system with antibodies, and can be fatal.

Common Allergy Triggers

The big question that always comes up when talking about allergies is why some people are predisposed to generate IgE antibodies to attack substances that are harmless to other people.

It is true that the origin of this immunological reaction remains a mystery, but it seems that there are some factors that favor this abnormal immune system behavior. One is genetic inheritance.

Another factor that influences immunological reactions is excessive or continuous exposure to a particular allergen, combined with the genetic predisposition of the individual.

There are other circumstances that seem to be of decisive importance in the origin of allergies: allergy precursors.

These are toxic substances or personal circumstances causing harm to our body and causing our immune system to become more sensitive to certain allergens and produce an allergic response.

Stress

It is proven that stress or strong emotions can exacerbate an allergic reaction or atopic dermatitis in people predisposed to allergies. The reactions originate in the allergy itself, but symptoms can be aggravated by heightened emotions and stressful situations.

Shock, depression, or anxiety can trigger allergic rhinitis or an asthma attack, for example, even when the patient has not come in contact with an allergen. This demonstrates how much our emotional state affects our physical health. Our body and mind, matter, and spirit are all interconnected.

The fact that emotional factors may trigger an allergy can make it difficult to trace the origin of the allergy in a person who is often in high-stress situations, who is frequently depressed, or who suffers from anxiety.

It is difficult to prevent stress and intense or negative emotions, but some self-help tools may assist in alleviating these problems. Yoga, reiki, Bach flowers, or tai-chi can be very effective in reducing episodes of anxiety, stress, and depression.

Environmental Pollution

As previously mentioned, allergies have significantly increased in industrialized countries over recent years.

Although allergies have been found in people for thousands of years, the fact is that the developed world has had a great impact on their presence. This can be partly explained if we consider that environmental pollution, specifically the particles derived from the combustion of diesel engines, are some of the main factors attributed to the increase in allergic sensitization of the urban population.

This has been demonstrated by clinical statistics that indicate that cases of allergies are more frequent in cities than in rural environments. This occurs even in pollen allergies, despite pollen being more prevalent in the countryside than in the city. This is also found in less developed countries, where allergies and asthma are almost nonexistent. In those areas, the causes of allergies are not genetic, because when residents move to industrialized countries, they tend to show allergic symptoms.

It has been proven that diesel particles attach to particles of pollen, and exponentially enhance their ability to cause allergies because it makes them much more irritating. This triggers inflammation, irritation, and increased permeability of the respiratory mucosa. These factors allow for the contaminated pollen proteins to enter our bodies more easily and trigger allergic reactions. Pollen is everywhere naturally, but it is the contaminated pollen that is the most harmful.

In addition to this issue, the polluted air of large cities is very irritating, causing our mucous to be sensitive to any stimulus, whether it is pollen, dust mites, or food, for example. People may be predisposed to allergies, but pollution helps trigger reactions by diminishing the quality of our physical condition.

Cigarette Smoke

Pollution does not only exist outside. In many cases, the interior of our home can become polluted due to various factors. Among these factors, the number one cause of indoor pollution is cigarette smoke. Numerous scientific studies show that exposure to cigarette smoke is associated in many cases with the development of allergies, among other diseases. This exposure affects more than just cigarette smokers; it also affects the people around them. The most heartbreaking example is of children who have been exposed to secondhand smoke who go on to develop asthma.

However, there are more reasons to refrain from smoking indoors than just preventing the development of allergies. If you live with someone who suffers from allergies, you should, by all means, avoid smoking in your home or car, as secondhand smoke also increases the likelihood of an allergic reaction. The best thing to do is to quit entirely, not only for your own health benefits, but also because the smoke particles attach themselves to clothing, skin, and hair. Even if you smoke outside, a large amount of smoke travels back inside with the smoker. There is evidence that smoke lingers for days in unventilated environments because the air does not dilute the irritating and toxic components that are attached to furniture, walls, ceilings, and floors. Filters and electronic air purifiers do not remove these harmful particles, because they cannot effectively remove the particles that are deposited on food, furniture, leather, clothing, and other surfaces.

If someone has smoked in a room, it can very easily trigger an asthma attack, rhinitis, or conjunctivitis in a person who suffers from allergies. This can happen even if the allergic person enters the room a day after anyone has smoked there.

Cigarette smoke is more damaging than one might first assume. It is not the nicotine that is addictive to the smoker. Cigarette smoke contains 443 known toxic carcinogens that are very harmful. These include tar, arsenic, cyanide, and carbon monoxide, among others. All of these generate free radicals in the body, which are unstable molecules that attack cells. The result is oxidation, aging of body tissues, and irritation and inflammation of mucous membranes. Therefore, both active and passive inhalation of cigarette smoke are among the worst players in the development of asthma, rhinitis, and sinusitis.

Change in Temperature

There are three ways in which a change in temperature, either cold to hot or vice versa, can affect people with allergies. It is essential, especially in cases of asthma and rhinitis, to avoid sudden temperature changes. Going out into the cold from a heated building in the winter is enough to cause an asthma attack, because the cold causes the bronchi to tighten, and this creates an almost immediate sensation of drowning. When you go outside, it is essential to wear warm clothing and a scarf that covers your nose and mouth to keep the air entering your lungs warm.

In the case of rhinitis, cold air can keep symptoms under control. Heated environments can dilate the nasal mucosa and start a sneezing fit or cause rhinorrhea (a runny nose). Try not to excessively heat your home, and avoid sudden temperature changes to prevent congestion in the upper respiratory tract.

Another factor that can trigger allergies is a change in weather. When it comes to weather, there are many different circumstances that can induce allergic reactions. Dry climates can trigger asthma, as can thunderstorms. On mildly rainy days, the rain can help clean pollen from the air, causing it to fall and stick to the wet ground. However, in the case of thunderstorms, the results are very different. The air we breathe is full of positive and negative ions. Prior to a thunderstorm, the levels of positive ions increase. Negative ions are generated mainly by water that evaporates into the air, either by rivers, waterfalls, or fountains. These ions are absorbed through the skin, and have beneficial effects in our bodies and respiratory systems, allowing for a greater absorption of oxygen, and purifying the air of dust and pollution. Excess positive ions in the air are harmful to people, animals, and plants. They can cause insomnia, depression, headaches, and bronchial problems. Positive ions are generated by the reaction between sunlight and the friction in the air, like wind or a storm. Many mothers of allergic children can predict a storm's arrival by the appearance of symptoms in their children.

There are also sources of positive ions in our homes, such as air pollution, air conditioning, electrical appliances, television screens and computers, and synthetic fibers, among others. To correct this electric imbalance in the air, and to clean it of impurities, we can use "ionizers," which are devices that generate negative ions and enhance the electrical composition of our atmosphere.

Ionizers and Their Benefits

There is no doubt that these devices affect the quality of the air we breathe, although no specific studies have been done on their impact on the households of allergic people. What is certain is that they produce negative ions and that these electrical particles have the following benefits:

- decrease the concentration of pathogenic germs in the air.
- decrease the concentration of allergens in the air, as these particles are electrically charged and deposited on the ground or on the surfaces of the furniture and walls and even inside the ionizer.
- give a sense of well being, improved mental performance, memory, and sleep, and above all, improve the status of asthmatic people.

Some of the appliances sold in the market produce ozone, so you should read the label carefully and buy an ionizer that does not release ozone.

Moreover, because it is an electric apparatus that generates an electromagnetic field with an approximately five-foot radius, you should not put it near people or keep it on for hours in places where people are working or sleeping, to avoid overloading the atmosphere with electromagnetic waves.

Lastly, a sudden change in temperature increases the possibility of suffering from cold urticaria, which can be very severe. This allergic reaction is caused by a sudden change in temperature when a person enters cold water after being in the sun for a while. Although hives may break out, this is not the worst issue. The real danger is the risk of dilation of blood vessels, resulting in hypotension and fainting. If the person who has it is alone, they could drown. Be careful to enter the water slowly, so that your body can adjust gradually to the temperature change. It is also recommended that you always swim with a companion in case you suffer an attack.

Dental Fillings

Fillings applied by dentists to fill the holes made by tooth decay are made of an amalgam of silver, mercury, aluminum, and copper. Although any excess metal is harmful to our bodies, the greatest risk is the presence of mercury. This metal is necessary in dental fillings because it creates the chemical reaction that hardens the filling once it is in place. The World Health Organization (WHO) said in 1977 that fillings release between three and seventeen milligrams of mercury into the body.

The problem gets worse if other metals are used in the mouth, like a bridge or other orthodontic appliances. This is because slight galvanic currents run between metals, accelerating the release of mercury ions, which travel through the lymphatic system to organs like the liver, the kidneys, and even the brain.

Symptoms that are shown in people with an allergy or sensitivity to mercury are depression, tremors, nervousness, memory loss, inability to concentrate, insomnia, cardiovascular disorders, and trembling legs. This can trigger other allergies like eczema, asthma attacks, and food allergies.

Environmental Factors

There are cases of allergic people who try conventional treatments and a long series of natural treatments without observing a significant improvement in their asthma or rhinitis. In these cases, the patient should consider the possibility that the problem is not caused by their body, but rather their home or work environment.

Rooms, houses, and buildings can be "sick," because of their location or orientation. This "disease" can come from elements such as where our house is located and the soil beneath it, or the orientation of our bed. Sleeping in the wrong place can be enough to cause insomnia, nightmares, psychosomatic diseases, and other problems sleeping.

The ancient Chinese science of feng shui investigates the energy relationship between a person and cosmo-telluric energy, which circulates under the floor and through the air. Other people like the Celts and certain African tribes also considered these energies, choosing locations for their sacred buildings based on geopathic-free places.

These factors are studied in not only feng shui. German scientist Dr. Hartmann studied the science of geobiology and came to similar conclusions. Water veins that run underground, telluric faults, the action of electromagnetic fields of the Earth—they are all factors that can interfere with both our mental and physical health. Telluric radiations (inside the earth) generate water veins or faults that can penetrate the thickest layers of metal and concrete. In fact, measurements to date show that the intensity is the same on the top floor of a skyscraper as it is on the ground floor, as it spreads vertically and can be enhanced by metal elements.

Hartmann created the modern science of geobiology, which is fully recognized in Sweden, Germany, Switzerland, France, Poland, and Russia, where prestigious geobiological research institutes have been in existence for over forty years. At present the new science of domobiotics that integrates geobiology, traditional and modern biobuilding, and feng shui is being incorporated in universities in Spain. Technical schools and colleges in Madrid, Valencia, Tenerife, Seville, and Barcelona investigate "sick buildings" and offer a new view of what makes a habitat healthy.

Technopathies. Additionally, current geophysical problems in the nature of our subsoils can be amplified if our home is also affected by other technological pathologies. The main cause of electromagnetic pollution comes from high and low frequency of electrical lines, computers, home appliances, and mobile telephones. Our body's energy is extremely sensitive to all sources of energy around it. If we sleep near a device connected to electricity, with a quartz watch, or on a spring mattress that alters the natural electromagnetic field, there are numerous factors that can cause distortions and regulations in all our bodily processes.

Diseases related to geopathies and technopathies

Upon initial exposure, one may often feel minor discomfort that is usually attributed to stress or life changes. However, as the length of exposure increases, it begins to affect the immune, endocrine, and hormonal systems. The loss of a healthy balance in our body can happen over the course of five years, on average. This results in many problems, depending on the sensitivity of each person. The pathologies are varied, but in most cases, it causes asthma, chronic bronchitis, and rhinitis as a result of the weakening of our immune system.

Other diseases that have been linked to households that had geopathies and technopathies are:

- Insomnia, sleep disorders, nightmares.
- Stress, aggressiveness, irritability.
- Distress, anxiety, bulimia.
- Psychophysical exhaustion, fatigue.
- Loss of appetite, anorexia.
- Depression.
- Loss of memory, lack of concentration.
- Respiratory disorders, rhinitis, sinusitis, bronchitis.
- Cardiovascular disorders, angina, myocardial infarction.
- Circulatory disorders, edema, varicose veins.
- Migraines, headaches.
- Eye-fatigue, myopia, presbyopia.
- Cataracts, retinopathy.
- Cervical, dorsal, lumbar pain.
- Rheumatism, gout, artosis, arthritis.

- Asthma, respiratory allergies.
- Cutaneous hypersensitivity, psoriasis.
- Psychic-Hypersensitivity, over-excitation, phobias.
- Vertigos, dizziness, spatial disorientation.
- Amenorrhea, dysmenorrhea, menstrual dysfunction.
- Impotence, anespermia, sterility.
- Abortions, congenital malformations.
- Metabolic dysfunction, goiter, diabetes.
- Leukemia, cancer.
- Immunodeficiencies, AIDS.
- Chromosomal aberrations, DNA abnormalities.

Allergic diseases: natural solutions

Asthma

Nowadays, asthma is a widespread disease. This could be because of an increase in environmental pollution, poor living habits, and allergies, but still many questions remain unanswered. For one, how come the list of asthma sufferers, especially children, is growing day by day in the industrialized world, while in rural areas, the numbers are maintained at the same level year after year?

What causes asthma? Among all allergic diseases, asthma is a chronic disease with the highest incidence in children. Most people know someone with asthma or a child with an allergy that produces it. Statistics say that in most industrialized countries, one in twenty adults and one in five children, that is, 5 to 20 percent respectively, suffer from asthma.

It is considered one of the most serious allergic diseases, because it can be disabling or even fatal. It has personal, familial, social, health, and economic repercussions.

Although not all people have allergic asthma, the most common cause of this disease is allergies. Studies have stated that all asthma cases are probably due to allergies, although the diagnostic methods currently available cannot always determine their origins, as there is a wide range of allergens that can trigger reactions.

It is difficult to define this disease exactly because it is a changing condition, whether in the types of patients or the types of crises in the same patient. What is known is that it is a chronic inflammatory lung disease that causes a narrowing of the airways. The consequence of this narrowing is that air does not circulate well in your lungs and the oxygen does not reach your alveoli and, therefore, does not reach your blood. Oxygen is essential for the proper functioning of every cell in your body, and without it, you may feel an unpleasant drowning sensation.

Unfortunately, anyone can develop asthma, from infants to adolescents. Asthma can be inherited, passed down from generation to generation within a family.

Asthma can be classified into two groups.

1. **Extrinsic:** Asthma caused by allergens. This type of asthma includes those cases in which IgE is present.
2. **Intrinsic:** Some cases are not caused by allergies, but occur during periods of stress or in patients with mood disorders. Among the most common are asthma associated with infectious processes, asthma induced by the presence of gastro-esophageal reflux, or asthma caused by continuous inhalation of irritating vapors. These diseases are associated with naso-sinusal polyposis and/or intolerance to nonsteroidal anti-inflammatory drugs (NSAIDs) such as aspirin, which trigger asthma attacks.

Extrinsic asthma is the most common kind of asthma and accounts for between 70 and 85 percent of all cases. It can be caused by inhalants, food, drugs, or insect bites.

Allergic asthma may, in turn, be divided into seasonal and perennial asthma, because of the cycle of allergen production, or due to foods that are eaten daily.

As we have explained above, there are a number of precursors that while not causing asthma, can trigger an attack in asthmatic individuals. For example, environmental pollutants like diesel particles, ozone, nitrous oxide, and sulfur compounds can lead to an asthmatic crisis. Also, pollution can increase the potency of some allergens, such as pollen, a factor that would explain why there are more people who suffer from allergies in cities than in rural areas, where in theory, there is more pollen in the air. In the city, these pollen particles are coated with a toxic layer from environmental pollution that makes them allergic "bombs."

Another precursor of a more potent allergy is cigarette smoke. There are more than four hundred toxic substances suspended in smoke that irritate the mucosa of the bronchi, which inhibits the respiratory function of asthmatic people. The danger is the same in people subjected to second-hand smoke as in smokers themselves. It is a powerful irritant that lasts for days, so it is advisable to not allow anyone to smoke in your home or car. Secondhand smoke also increases the chances of children to develop asthma, as it irritates their airways.

Other products also have harmful effects on the lining of our airways when inhaled, such as detergents, household cleaners, bleach, and ammonia. These are strong irritants, and it is recommended that you check your labels because many cleaners contain ammonia. Ideally, use neutral cleaning products, as many scents trigger reactions as well.

Among the many other asthma triggers are viral or bacterial respiratory infections, paints, solvents, food additives such as dyes or preservatives, wood smoke, formaldehyde, strong perfumes, hyperventilation, menstrual factors, aspirin, and other drugs.

There is also exercise-induced asthma, which is triggered by physical activity such as sports. If you are in the habit of exercising, this may cause your airways to close up, especially if you start suddenly, or are in a cold environment. When one breathes normally, the nasal mucosa warms the air before it reaches the pulmonary alveoli, but when you exercise, you inhale greater volumes of air than normal, and your nose cannot adequately heat this much air.

The cold air then reaches your bronchial mucosa, and that can cause local alterations in your hypersensitive bronchi and lead to asthma attacks. It is therefore necessary that you avoid exercising outdoors early in the morning or late in the afternoon during the winter, but if you do, protect your nose and mouth well to prevent the entry of cold air into your bronchi.

Asthma, a disease with a long history

Although asthma research has begun to pay off recently, the truth is that this disease has hampered the breathing of many people for thousands of years.

The first historical reference made to asthmatic symptoms dates back to ancient Egypt, where some 3,500 years ago it was mentioned in the Ebers Papyrus.

A thousand years later, Hippocrates described the symptoms again and named the disease "asthma," meaning, "panting breath." His historical references also lead us to the time of the Roman Emperor Trajan at the beginning of our era, where it was described as a mysterious disease that was associated with exercise and that came and went without notice.

The first detailed description came from the pen of Galen, the personal physician of Emperor Marcus Aurelius. And in the tenth century, another royal physician, Maimonides, also mentioned it in his writings.

Over the following centuries asthma was studied by Paracelsus, Thomas Willis, and Thomas Sidenham, among others, until the seventeenth century when the first book on asthma was written, where its cause was assigned to laughter, emotional stress, exercise, and respiratory infections.

➤

In the nineteenth century, the French doctor Laennec, with the help of a stetho-scope, was able to provide the first accurate description of asthma, with more information providing more characteristics of this respiratory disease over recent decades.

Although research has advanced greatly, the exact cause of asthma is still unkown, and the rest of the history of this research remains unwritten.

What are the symptoms of asthma? People with asthma suffer from chronic inflammation of the bronchi, even when they are apparently well. This constant swelling of the face and the bronchi produces what doctors call "bronchial hyperreactivity," that is, a disproportionate reaction against a range of stimuli that are usually harmless to the general population, producing bronchial contraction.

All asthma sufferers' airways are hypersensitive or hyperreactive to certain stimuli, but the triggers vary from one person to another. Among the most common are exercise, allergies, viral infections, and smoke. The hypersensitive lining of the inside of the bronchi reacts to a certain trigger and becomes inflamed and swollen and begins producing mucous. As a result, the muscles lining the swollen airways tighten and contract, causing the airways to become even more narrow and blocked.

Asthma produces the following symptoms: coughing, wheezing, and dyspnea. The cough is usually dry at first, and after a few days becomes productive, that is, with secretions. Wheezing is a whistling sound in the chest that can be painful and sometimes can be heard without the aid of a stethoscope. Dyspnea, or difficulty breathing, is fatigue, a feeling of choking or breathlessness, which can feel like drowning. All this is caused by a narrowing of the diameter of the bronchi, which slows the passage of air.

All these symptoms can occur simultaneously or separately. In addition, they can vary greatly from one patient to another in intensity, frequency, and duration, even varying in the same patient at different times. Typically they manifest intermittently with symptom-free periods, although there are also cases of patients who suffer symptoms constantly and daily. To further complicate the situation, the symptoms can show up suddenly, even over just a few minutes, or gradually over several days, and they are usually worse at night.

Treatment. As you may have read, or maybe learned by experience, asthma is a serious ailment and requires close collaboration between the physician or therapist and the patient to improve the condition of the patient's bronchi and to avoid future crises. When seeking conventional or alternative medical treatments, it is essential to do so under the supervision of specialists, and for the patient to take responsibility for their health in order to have the most success. The patient needs to follow the treatment strictly and avoid any contact with allergens that cause asthma.

Bear in mind that an asthma attack requires immediate intervention. Do not hesitate to resort to drugs or conventional medicine if you feel unwell. Both methods—conventional and alternative—offer solutions in cases of allergies, and it is up to the patient to find whether one or the other, or a combination of the two, will help treat the allergies. However, it is essential to maintain clear communication with your physician or therapist and keep them abreast of what you are taking, as there may be complications when taking different medicines at once, like drugs and herbal infusions, for example. Herbal medicines have powerful active ingredients that must be taken into account when taking bronchodilators or anti-inflamatory drugs. Explain to your specialists what you drink, what you take, and how you feel physically and mentally.

CONVENTIONAL MEDICINE

Asthma has been present in the history of mankind for millennia, and there are many remedies that have been tested to try to cure or mitigate its adverse effects on the health and quality of life of asthmatics. However, it wasn't until the 1980s that a better understanding of asthma's origin and treatments was achieved.

It has been found that modern environmental conditions have led to an increase in allergic asthma in patients, and, even worse, a higher incidence of severe cases. Allopathic medicine, which considers asthma to be a chronic disease, uses several treatments that can help patients lead a more or less normal life, with some unavoidable side effects.

Specialists try to diagnose the source of the illness through observing the patient's physical symptoms and running medical tests. They also usually ask the patient to keep a written diary of symptoms, including all emotional and environmental factors that could be causing their asthma attacks.

Upon diagnosing the patient with asthma, the doctor will prescribe two types of palliative medicine: rescue medications and controller medications, also known as preventative or maintenance medications.

Rescue, or symptomatic, medications work immediately to relieve asthma symptoms once they occur. They dilate the bronchi, reduce inflammation and mucous, and open up the airways. They are usually administered orally, via injection, or by inhaler. Although these medications relieve symptoms almost immediately, they do not work in the long-term, or prevent asthma attacks.

Two types of medications are prescribed:
- quick-acting bronchodilators.
- intravenous or oral corticosteroids.

In order to avoid a relapse, anti-inflammatory control or maintenance drugs are prescribed. Their purpose is to restore the

123

condition of the bronchi and reduce inflammation in the airways. These treatments are taken over long periods of time, even for years.

Among the various kinds of control medications are the following:

- inhaled steroids to prevent inflammation.
- leukotriene inhibitors.
- long-acting bronchodilators.
- cromolyn sodium or nedocromil sodium.
- aminophylline or theophylline.
- combination of anti-inflammatory drugs and bronchodilators.

Conventional medicine has a third tool: immunotherapy. In this case, the goal is not to prevent or alleviate the symptoms, but to solve the problem that causes asthma. This treatment, known as "allergy shots," has been recognized by the World Health Organization as an effective method in the cure of asthma.

The purpose of these shots is to have the body develop a tolerance to the allergen and "get used to" it in order to no longer recognize it as a harmful substance. For the treatment to take effect it is essential to know that it is not always easy to trace the source of the allergy, and that the patient can be allergic to one protein at a time (mites, pollen, etc.). Immunotherapy yields strong results after several years of treatment.

This treatment has been proven effective in children, although it is possible that they can outgrow their allergies due to physical changes that accompany adolescence.

NATURAL THERAPIES

Many asthma sufferers have experienced significant improvements in their symptoms through alternative treatments and natural therapies. The range in treatments is vast and patient preferences play an important role in deciding on pursuing one or more of them.

Complementary methods and their effects are more potent when acting in synergy. For example, acupuncture can be very effective, but that power increases if the patient follows a natural diet based on healthy foods, free of sugar and dairy.

- **Natural Diet**

  A healthy diet free of additives, fats, and dairy may not only be helpful but essential to the health of asthma sufferers. Avoiding particular allergy-inducing proteins can help the body fight symptoms of asthma and boost the immune system and the body's overall health. A healthy body needs a healthy diet, and eating mindfully and with proper guidelines will help you achieve the balance you need.

  Naturopathy provides specific dietary guidelines to prevent asthma and relieve symptoms. Some specialists also recommend occasional fasting to detoxify the body, which should always be done under their supervision.

  The ideal diet for anyone should consist largely of plant-based whole foods. This is also recommended for asthmatic people, who should also avoid allergens in case of developing allergic asthma. Remember that a small amount of an allergen is enough to trigger a crisis and you must have the willpower to completely remove them from your diet, however much you like the particular food, whether it is milk, chocolate, nuts, or other triggers.

  In the case of people with asthma, it is recommended to reduce the consumption of garlic, onion, and citrus in order to decrease the development of mucous, and to clear the bronchi and intestine. For this reason you should also avoid all dairy products from cows, and sugar, which are all great generators of mucous.

  Recent studies have found that people with asthma have a low level of blood sugar and a high level of potassium, so eating salty foods is discouraged. Moreover, asthma attacks usually occur in the early hours of the morning, when blood sugar levels are lowest. Drinking a few tablespoons of sugar diluted in a glass of water can help temporarily relieve symptoms.

The main "ingredient" in the diet of an asthmatic person is antioxidants. They are a group of vitamins, minerals, and enzymes that come from our diet and protect us from free radicals that relentlessly attack our immune system and our body. Free radicals are the agents responsible for the hardening and swelling of tissues, such as the bronchi in asthma. They come from exposure to radiation and toxic chemical agents, overexposure to the sun's rays, and various metabolic processes. One of their most harmful effects is to accelerate the aging process.

The main sources of antioxidants in our diets are sprouted grains, fruits, and vegetables. The most powerful are vitamins (A, B, C, and E), beta-carotene, and certain minerals, such as selenium and magnesium. But the list is very extensive and you should consume plenty of fruits and fresh vegetables. Another star is fish for its high levels of omega-3 fatty acids, which have a recognized anti-inflammatory effect. Fish also provide B vitamins that help fight stress and inflammation. The following foods and drinks can provoke an asthma attack even when the patient does not suffer from a food allergy:

— Food and beverages containing chemical additives such as sulfites and sulfur dioxides: prepared salads, chips, wine, beer, dried fruit, and most processed foods containing sulfites or metabisulfite dyes E220 to E227, which are not always indicated on the label.

— Foods that produce stomach acid.

— Alcoholic drinks can cause contractions in the airways, as can beverages containing caffeine such as coffee, tea, and some sodas .

— Foods that release histamine: seafood, cured cheeses, meat, red wine, yeast, tomatoes, spinach, strawberries, bananas, pineapple, eggplant, sausage, nuts, eggs, and canned food.

— Some asthmatics do not tolerate the aroma of cooked food and even just the smell of hot food on their plate can trigger a reaction in some extreme cases.

- **Homeopathy**

Homeopathy is one of the therapies that achieve better results in the treatment of allergies. Treatments are long-term, and use the doctrine of "like cures like" to treat symptoms and help the body learn to tolerate allergens. The prescribed remedies take into account the physical constitution, character, and other personal data of the patient.

This treatment is very personalized and requires the diagnosis of a trained professional. The ultimate goal is to boost your immune system in order to improve its response so you can avoid allergic reactions caused by IgE and histamine release.

However, there are some "first aid" remedies that can lend a hand when symptoms occur. Below are some examples:

Coccus cacti: for spasmodic cough with abundant mucous of viscous texture.

Arsenic-D30: relieves severe asthma attack when it occurs between midnight and three in the morning. The attack is accompanied by fear and anxiety, breathlessness, and a continuous cough.

— *Ipecacuanha*: for excess mucous

— *Tartarus emeticus*: for diarrhea, loss of color in face, and impending pneumonia.

— *Teucrium*: for severe allergies in autumn.

— *Sulfuricum-Natrium*: for asthma in a home or very humid region; aggravation caused by rain or fog.

— *Ambra ignatia*: for asthma caused by sadness and anxiety.

● Phytotherapy

Herbs offer palliative solutions in cases of allergic asthma. Pharmaceutical laboratories have succeeded in synthesizing many of the active ingredients in herbs to create medications. However, plants contain many other elements in addition to the active ingredient, and using them in their natural forms ultimately provides natural and balanced solutions for your body without side effects.

Taking an infusion may sound silly, but it is very good for your health. Consult your herbalist to find an herbal plant or mixture that suits you and your method of preparation of herbal tea.

Herbalist's Advice

If you suffer from allergies, you should always consult an herbalist and never take herbal medicines on your own.

Although plants have no side effects, if you are allergic to grasses, you may not be able to consume a tisane of corn; or chamomile or dandelion if your allergy is caused by the pollen of composite plants.

Choose an experienced herbalist, who thoroughly understands the disease and knows how to advise on allergy treatments.

Take a break with a steaming cup of tea and while you drink it, focus on all the good elements contributing to the health of your bronchi. Remember that your mind has great healing effects on your body.

We'll show you some of the herbs commonly used in cases of allergic asthma, but remember that expert advice is always necessary.

Chinese Angelica	For cases of hay fever, mites, and animal dander. Steep the dried roots in boiling water for thirty minutes. Have one cup after each meal.
Coleus	The extract of this Ayurvedic herb has been shown in recent clinical studies in Germany to dilate the bronchial tubes almost as effectively as with conventional medication. Inhale steam from hot water with a few drops of extract added to it, or take fifteen drops of extract in a half glass of water per day.
Ephedra	Very suitable for all allergic conditions. It is a potent bronchodilator and should always be taken with the advice of a good expert.
Echinacea	Widely used for asthma treatment. It is non-allergenic and has anti-inflammatory properties and stimulates the defenses.
Chinese Skullcap	Possesses anti-inflammatory properties due to its high content of bioflavonoids.
Euphorbia	Very useful for chronic asthma due to its anti-spasmodic effect.
Gingko	Relieves asthma, persistent cough, and nasal congestion.
Lobelia	Used in combination with various herbs to treat asthma due to its antispasmodic properties and levels of guaifenesin.
Chamomile	Its antispasmodic and sedative properties may be useful in asthma attacks.
Licorice	Well-known anti-inflammatory and allergenic properties.
Coltsfoot	Exerts mucolytic and expectorant agents.

Also, you can prepare herbal syrups for coughs caused by asthma and spasmodic bronchitis by combining various plants. Mix plantain, coltsfoot, thyme, fennel, and lemon balm. Put two tablespoons of the mixture into a container and pour a quart of boiling water over the mixture. Let stand ten minutes, strain, and add honey to sweeten. Take three to five cups a day.

● **Acupuncture**

Acupuncture is an ancient therapy that is part of traditional Chinese medicine. It involves the insertion of needles into specific body points or acupoints. The location of these points is very important and they are distributed over twelve meridians or vital energy channels.

Each meridian is connected to a specific organ and each point has a specific action.

Of all the therapies of traditional Chinese medicine, acupuncture is the most widely spread in the West. Its goal is to achieve balance in the body by treating the root of the problem, which may take time. However, this therapy is an effective treatment for many diseases, especially chronic illnesses.

It has been approved by the World Health Organization as an effective therapy for many health disorders, including asthma.

To control chronic asthma, the meridians and acupoints that regulate and boost the immune system defenses are targeted. In addition, the meridians linked to the lungs, kidneys, and spleen are also targeted to eliminate mucous and bronchial congestion by reducing moisture in the body.

A minimum of fifteen to twenty sessions on a weekly basis are necessary to achieve effects. When administering acupuncture to children, laser needles or moxa are used. Smaller needles are best for treating children.

● **Aromatherapy**

This therapy uses the scents of essential oils extracted from plants to achieve physical and emotional well-being. The oils can be applied to the skin or added to bath water, inhalers, or incense burners. Its active ingredients enter your body through the skin and lymphatic system and are then transported to all organs of our body. They also reach the olfactory bulb, which lies in front of the hypothalamus and is responsible for our emotions.

Some of the most commonly used essential oils are eucalyptus, hyssop, lavender, frankincense, lemon balm, thyme, anise, rosemary, pine, and cypress. You should not breathe in the oils in hot vapors, because they are moister and might overload your bronchi.

A specialist can recommend to you certain essential oils that you can add to almond oil and use during a massage. A chest massage in a warm environment using these oils can greatly relieve symptoms and treat allergies.

● **Reflexology**

The feet and hands contain reflex points linked to all organs of the body, including the lungs. Reflexology is based on targeting these reflex points through massaging our feet and our hands.

A simple massage can soothe and relax you, but when using massage as treatment for allergies, it is recommended that you go to a specialist. Working the right areas can reduce your stress and relieve your bronchi. The reflex points of the lungs are located on the balls of your feet, and in the case of the hands they are only on the right hand, on the palm of the hand, below the knuckles. You can massage them daily to help you in your recovery.

● **Compresses and Poultices**

Remedies like these may seem antiquated, but they work. The heat on your skin, combined with the base of the poultice, allow its benefits to travel through your nervous system via your skin pores, thus getting to the root of your problem.

They are simple remedies that usually provide almost immediate relief, if only for a few hours. Sometimes, simple solutions can be more effective than something more extreme.

Lemon juice helps to reverse the process of bronchial contraction. Our grandmothers already knew that if you put a cotton or linen cloth soaked in pure lemon juice around the entire thorax, this will help you breathe better. The wet part is placed in contact with the skin and you can leave it on for as long as you want.

Curd compresses are also effective.

Wrap a layer of cheese curds in gauze or thin cotton fabric. Place on the chest and cover with a towel.

- **Breathing Exercises**

There are specific methods of breathing in and out slowly that will help strengthen the lungs. While this will not cure asthma, they are useful because they help control breathing and could be very helpful during an acute asthma attack.

When an attack is coming, one should breathe calmly, but anxiety makes patients feel short of breath and they may try to inhale as much air as possible into their congested lungs. Some professionals advise that during an attack, the patient should inhale slowly through the nose, hold his/her breath for a few seconds (to allow the air to fill the lungs), and exhale slowly.

This should relax the muscles and keep tension from pinching the thorax. Learn to relax your shoulders and abdominal area while breathing slowly with the diaphragm. This can improve lung performance, and increase air intake.

There are many breathing and relaxation therapies that provide very important tools for asthmatic patients.

Buteyko

This breathing method was created by the Russian scientist K. P. Buteyko after years of working with people affected by respiratory diseases. Hospitals in Russia practiced the technique, and the government recognized its effective results in 1980.

The World Health Organization states that a healthy adult at rest breathes four to six liters of air per minute. K. P. Buteyko's research corroborates this estimate. But his research on breathing found that in a hundred thousand people suffering from various diseases, all breathed in excess; some group consumed an air volume three, four, or even five times higher than normal. In the wake of this research, Buteyko considered asthma and many other diseases, due to the common symptom of bad breath. He found hyperventilation as a result of excessive breathing involved, therefore indicating a CO_2 deficiency in the body. All asthma sufferers have chronic hyperventilation.

Patients learn to practice a few sessions of reduced respiration per day, that is, a gradual reduction in the volume of air. This technique is effective, but to get the best results you have to make time for it every day, in three or four half-hour sessions daily. When this technique is mastered, you can practice it while doing other activities such as reading, working, or walking.

It is also recommended to combine this method of reduction with other beneficial breathing techniques for asthma, such as meditation, yoga, or relaxation.

Respiratory Psychotherapy

This breathing technique is to remove physical and energetic blockages that inhibit breathing. To do this, you must become aware of the way you breathe. That is, learn how to make a conscious breath.

This is achieved through practicing a series of breathing techniques that remove blockages and reveal the existence of our true Self.

We have seen that the emotional status of a person plays a very important role in asthma. Respiration is a process that can help both physical and emotional problems.

When a person is involved in a conflict or a negative emotional situation, respiratory muscles contract (especially the solar plexus) and form a muscular armor that restricts the free flow of air. Respiratory psychotherapy helps the practitioner become aware of these contractions and release them.

The techniques used by the respiratory psychotherapy are therapeutic bioenergetics and respiration. The goal is for us to realize how we breathe and help us discover our physical and emotional blocks: know how to ease tensions that cause difficulty breathing.

- **Reiki**

In the case of allergies, including asthma, our body turns harmless substances into enemies. Reiki, an energy therapy of Japanese origin, helps strengthen the immune system by correcting your body and mind's energy imbalance. It can first relieve symptoms, alleviating congestion and soothing irritation, and then help heal the whole body to avoid future reactions, focusing on the source of the allergy. Teachers impart healing by reaching the Self and restoring your source of energy. All you need to do is channel energy through the teacher's hands, and feel their support.

Although it may seem unbelievable or exaggerated, more and more people are turning to this therapy as a treatment for a number of ailments. In fact, it is used in hospitals and by emergency response teams like firefighters and police.

Yoga

Yoga has been practiced since the dawn of time and has been proven effective for millennia. This movement therapy is based on breathing and stretching postures that increase airflow, so it is very suitable for people with asthma to help relieve their symptoms and reverse its adverse effects.

With its continued practice the lungs expand, the chest muscles relax, and the levels of vital energy are increased through relaxation and increased oxygen intake. These factors are of great importance when it comes to managing an asthma attack because knowing how to relax and control breathing helps reduce the feeling of panic that often causes people to seize up during acute asthmatic crisis.

In cases where asthma is triggered by emotional circumstances, yoga is a wonderful tool that helps to find inner peace through meditation and relaxation, which decreases anxiety and improves self-esteem.

Its benefits are also recognized by conventional medicine, and hospitals recommend it as therapy for asthmatics. Daily practice helps you achieve good results by reducing bronchial inflammation and histamine levels, and helping to find emotional balance. It is also good therapy for children, and they can practice with their parents.

The postures or asanas recommended for asthma sufferers are chest-opening exercises, such as triangle pose, cobra, and bow; inverted poses like candle; and backbends like fish and supine pelvic tilts.

The breathing exercises practiced in yoga are very beneficial because they teach practitioners how to breathe effectively and deeply. The rapid abdominal breathing stimulates the tissues of the lungs, relaxes chest muscles, and provides energy to the body. Alternating respiration is calming and, if practiced along with meditation, brings harmony and peace to the patient.

Allergic Rhinitis or Hay Fever

Rhinitis is one of the most common allergic conditions. Its symptoms may not be severe, and the quality of life of people who suffer from this allergy can be affected for short periods out of the year, or chronically.

This immune disorder, also called "hay fever," causes an exaggerated response of the mucosa in the nasal passages from inhaling pollen or other allergens. Sneezing, runny nose, watery eyes, congestion, and headaches are annoying symptoms that accompany this reaction and may occur at any age.

The rising population of allergic people has increased awareness of this illness. It's important to take into account both the professional and personal environments of the patient when treating the source of the allergy. Rhinitis affects the quality of life of patients, who feel as though they have a perpetual cold for weeks, or even all year.

What causes allergic rhinitis? As in the case of asthma, rhinitis is a respiratory condition that is triggered by the inhalation of airborne allergens.

When an allergic person is in an environment with pollen, dust mites, mold, or other airborne allergens, these allergens trigger the body to start making IgE, which in turn releases histamine, causing the lining of the nose, throat, and sinuses to become inflamed.

This starts a bout of strong and uncontrollable sneezing; nasal congestion, and resulting headaches; constant, runny, clear, watery, mucous; itchy, watery eyes; fatigue; irritability; and a huge supply of handkerchiefs.

Although called "hay fever," the fact is that it is not just the pollen from hay that causes allergies in certain people. Many others, such as pollens of grasses, herbs, trees, shrubs, and flowers, make spring and summer a real ordeal for those with rhinitis. If allergy testing determines that pollen is the source of the allergy, this causes seasonal rhinitis that only occurs at the time of pollination of the plant in question.

However, there are other allergens that can cause allergic rhinitis continuously in the daily life of the affected person. The most common are mites, mold, and animal dander, causing what medicine calls "perennial" or "chronic" rhinitis. The reaction may begin immediately upon contact with the allergens, but late-phase reactions also occur due to constant contact with triggers. In these cases, it is difficult to identify the causative allergen because there is no clear cause-effect reaction. For example, in the case of a child with rhinitis caused by a dog's dander, the child may pet and play with the dog without sneezing, but suffer an attack hours later. The origin of some late reactions can only be uncovered if allergy tests are positive, because there is no clear evidence to help us find the cause.

Unfortunately, there are a few occasions when people obtain negative results after testing for rhinitis. It then is called unexplained allergic rhinitis. Allergy sufferers should ideally avoid the allergens causing their reactions, but if these allergens remain unidentified, the patient's symptoms will persist relentlessly.

Sometimes a food intolerance, rather than an allergen, can cause the same symptoms as rhinitis, but it is a pseudoallergy and not an allergic reaction. Diagnostic testing for intolerances to foods and food additives may yield results where allergy tests came up negative. Also, even without suffering from a specific intolerance or allergy to dairy products, dairy should be eliminated from your diet if you have rhinitis, as dairy causes the production of excess mucous. This causes hypersensitivity not only in the intestines, but also in the bronchi, skin, and nose.

In addition, being stressed, sad, or scared can also trigger an attack. Psycho-emotional circumstances have a significant impact on our immune system. Stressful or annoying situations can cause a "lowering of defenses," and give rise to a series of reactions like sneezing and other symptoms.

Cigarette smoke can also trigger reactions once the mucous is irritated, even hours or days after being exposed to the smoke. You should not allow smoking in your home or your car if you suffer from rhinitis, because it is very likely that the smoke will cause an attack.

How do the symptoms manifest? Rhinitis begins with a slight tingling in the nose that quickly turns into a barrage of severe sneezing. These sneezing fits are so intense that the patient may not even get a word in between sneezes. Next, the patient develops a runny, red nose; itchy, watery eyes; runny, watery mucous; and a nasal voice. There are also unseen symptoms like headaches, itchy throat, sinus pressure, sore throat, fatigue, moodiness, and insomnia.

The nose normally produces a liquid substance that is commonly called a "runny nose." The liquid is clear and watery, and helps prevent dust, bacteria, viruses, and allergens from reaching the lungs. It is usually not very noticeable, and is only produced in a small amount. However, in people with rhinitis, mucosal irritation in the nose produces higher levels of this liquid, and causes it to become thicker as well. It can flow both out of the nose and down the back of the throat, which causes coughing. This increase in nasal secretion in the throat is called "postnasal drip."

Why does the nose become irritated? When the allergens enter the nose, the immunoglobulin IgE alerts mast cells of the intruders, and they release histamine. This substance inflames the lining of the sinuses, nose, and throat. This can be confused with the symptoms of pertussis, especially in children when the pharyngeal ring is inflamed.

In certain individuals, allergies produce over years what is called an "allergic march," when the IgE that is released in the mucous "travels" to other parts of the body, such as the skin or the bronchi. This explains the cases of rhinitis that end up further complicating dermatitis or asthma. At other times, the pollen ingested acts on the intestinal mucosa and causes cramps and diarrhea. Rhinitis should be treated with great importance.

A person can also have allergic rhinitis not triggered by allergens. In this case the condition may occur as a side effect of the continuous use of topical nasal sprays that produce a rebound effect. One may apply nasal drops to clear nasal congestion from a cold, but if these drops are used daily for a long period and then discontinued, the mucosa of the nose and sinuses tend to swell when the effects of the drug dissipate. If more doses are applied, the mucosa becomes even more inflamed and a vicious cycle begins as the body adjusts to the new dosage and requires more doses more frequently to relieve symptoms.

Rhinitis can also be produced by hormonal changes or modifications in the structure of the nose, as with a deviated septum or the growth of nasal polyps.

Finally, there is also infectious rhinitis, which is nothing but the congestion and runny nose caused by the common cold. The virus that causes an infection occurs in the mucous membranes of the nose and sinuses.

Treatment. In the case of allergic rhinitis, the patient should above all avoid the allergen causing the reaction. However, the underlying problem is often caused by stress and poor diet, leading to a weak immune system and sickness. These are the real reasons that certain people have an exaggerated response to substances that are innocuous to most others.

Conventional medicine treats the symptoms, whereas natural medicine treats the causes of these symptoms. It is up to you to decide which method to pursue for treatment, but we strongly recommend that you try to solve the problem at its source.

Treating yourself with natural therapies will help restore your balance.

CONVENTIONAL MEDICINE

First of all, a doctor should prescribe all medicines you take, and you should never self-medicate. The health of your body is a very serious thing and you should act responsibly, so if you decide on conventional medicine, be sure to visit a good allergist who thoroughly understands your condition and knows which treatments can help you.

Of all the drugs that allergists prescribe, antihistamines are most commonly used to control the symptoms of rhinitis. These drugs counteract the symptoms produced by histamine, but one of its main side effects is drowsiness, which makes it impossible to carry on a normal lifestyle. However, medicine has designed some antihistamines that do not usually cause drowsiness in most cases. Nevertheless, when you stop taking antihistamines and then come into contact with the allergen, the symptoms will reappear with the same force as before, as the drugs only treat the symptoms and do not prevent future reactions.

Another effective medication is corticosteroid nasal spray. It is applied directly to the nasal mucosa and eliminates nasal congestion. These steroids are not related to anabolic steroids used by some athletes to improve their performance.

If the origin of the allergy can be traced to a single allergen, the patient may be treated with vaccine immunotherapy. The treatment can take a long time, but has good results.

NATURAL THERAPIES

There are a large number of options in natural medicine that can not only help you control your rhinitis as effectively as conventional medicine, but, in addition, may prevent the reappearance of symptoms and, in some cases, help you overcome rhinitis entirely.

The synergy that occurs between two or more therapies can increase the benefits of these treatments.

- **Natural Diet**

Nutritionists recommend a diet based on fresh, plant-based foods, with a large amount of fresh fruits and vegetables so that your body receives high levels of vitamins, beta-carotene, and bioflavonoids that help keep the inflammation under control and return strength to your immune system. You should avoid foods that contain a high content of histamine to prevent mucosal inflammatory agents from overcharging. These foods include chocolate, eggs, cheese, tomatoes, pineapple, strawberries, nuts, fish, shellfish, and citrus.

In addition, you should avoid food additives because they can also generate an intolerance or an allergic response. These are mostly found in refined products such as commercial baked goods, prepared food, and packaged food.

In the chapter on allergens, we provide a full list of the chemical additives commonly used in the food industry today. In cases of allergic rhinitis, you should completely eliminate mucous-forming foods such as dairy products and sugar from your diet to avoid overloading your mucous membranes and intestines. Also avoid coffee and alcohol, as they do not provide any nutritional benefit, but quite the opposite. It is also highly advisable that you increase your fluid intake because it will help reduce congestion. You can drink infusions of herbal medicines to help further relieve your symptoms after a crisis. Soups, broths, fruit and vegetable juices, or nut-based milks are other great options. These fluids provide vitamins, energy, and wellness to your tired body, which has been subjected to extra wear. Naturopaths recommend carrot, cucumber, and parsley juices for their powerful detoxifying effects on your body.

On the other hand, you can improve the state of your immune system by increasing your consumption of garlic and onions, which contain quercetin, a potent anti-inflammatory agent. Pumpkin is also very beneficial because it provides a lot of beta-carotene during the fall and winter, when there is a limited selection of fruits and vegetables. Honey also provides many benefits. Experts recommend taking a tablespoon every morning to boost the immune system. Although sold in many varieties and textures, it is best that you buy local, artisanal honey. Because local honey will be made from the flowers in your area, you can ingest small amounts of these pollens and help your body get used to their proteins, helping you to react less and less. As always, seek advice from your nutritionist before making any decisions, including taking honey, if you suffer from hay fever or some food allergies, to avoid any undesirable effects.

Chewing honeycomb is also recommended in the winter. You can chew honeycomb as many times per day as you want and it will help your sinuses stay clear. Treat it as you would chewing gum, and chew it for a quarter of an hour at a time, leaving at least an hour between each time.

- **Homeopathy**

In the case of allergic asthma, homeopathy shows excellent results in patients with rhinitis by balancing our bodies both physically and emotionally in order to combat the disease globally.

Suffice it to say, you should avoid as much contact as possible with substances that provoke your allergies, at least until your body is completely restored. Also, do not try to gradually adapt to the allergen yourself, as this can worsen allergic conditions and increase your symptoms' intensity.

Ideally, the homeopath will be able to prescribe a remedy that is suitable for your allergy. However, it is not always easy to find the right remedy at first, since physical and emotional data can get mixed up.

Certain homeopathic methods prescribe an initial dose of a remedy that produces what is called "similar aggravation." This is an intensification of the patient's existing symptoms. If it occurs, it means that the remedy is correct. This process takes time, but the treatments have good results. Look for a homeopath that you completely trust and follow their instructions to the letter. You must remember you both are on the same path in search of your self-healing.

There are some homeopathic remedies that can also help you cope with allergic rhinitis outbreaks:

— The most common remedies are Luffa operculata and Allium

— For a runny nose and watery eyes: 6C dilutions of Arsenicum album, Euphrasia, Natrum muriatricum, Nux vomica, and Kali iodatum.

— For thick mucous: 6C dilutions of Calcium Sulphate and Hepar Sulphur.

● **Physiotherapy**

Helichrysum	Helichrysum is a potent anti-inflammatory that gives excellent results in controlling outbreaks of sneezing and inflammation of the mucosa, relieves itching, and stops a runny nose. It is sold in health centers in the form of syrup.
Mullein	Curbs post-nasal drips. Put the leaves in boiling water, and, leaning over to inhale the vapors, cover your head with a towel to keep the steam around your face.
Elder	Known for its anti-inflammatory properties.

Licorice	A root and a potent antiallergenic that has been used for thousands of years.
Plantain	Relieves excess mucous.
Chamomile	Relieves puffy eyes. After brewing chamomile, soak two cotton balls in the infusion, and then lay them over your eyes for ten minutes.
Fenugreek	Helps prevent attacks. If you have hay fever, you should start taking it a few days before pollination begins.
Ephedra	Contains the active ingredient in a popular antihistamine medication, ephedrine. The herbalist should tell you the exact dosage because if abused, ephedra accelerates the heart rate and blood pressure.
Myrtle	Relieves nasal congestion. Irrigate each nostril with this using a syringe or plastic bulb.
Echinacea	This herb boosts the immune system, which is always helpful for people with allergies. If your rhinitis is seasonal, take echinacea a few weeks before pollination to help prevent attacks.
Stinging Nettle	Reduces the secretion of mucous.

● **Acupuncture**

This ancient therapy has proven very effective in cases of allergic rhinitis. Not only can targeting specific acupoints help reduce inflammation, but it also boosts the immune system and cleans blockages in your body's energy channels. Acupuncturists often work the meridians for the liver, large intestine, or the lungs, although the diagnosis of each patient is completely personalized, so the treatment may vary.

The needles can sometimes produce pain, especially in certain troublesome acupoints used to treat rhinitis. These points are located on both sides of the nostrils and eye-brows, and the tops of the earlobes. If it is too painful, the therapist can stimulate these points with a laser instead of a needle. In this case, the effects will not be as great, but the session will be more bearable.

Natural therapies treat the body with the most respect, and though symptoms are resolved quickly, the treatments require repeated sessions to get to the root of the condition. A patient should schedule weekly acupuncture sessions of about a half hour in length until the patient shows improvement, whereupon the sessions can become less frequent.

- **Aromatherapy**

Essential oils can also provide relief for your sinuses. Lavender essential oil, when applied with a gentle massage under the eyes, can clear nasal congestion. Inhaling a few drops of essential oil of lemon balm, lavender, chamomile, or eucalyptus can also help. Do not use chamomile oil if you are pregnant.

The vapors from hot water with two or three drops of sandalwood or pine oils added to it can be a very effective nasal decongestant. Niaouli is another effective oil, but not recommended in children because it can provoke a bronchospasm.

- **Oligotherapy**

The body requires trace elements of certain essential minerals that are essential to biological processes such as the synthesis of hormones, digestion, cell reproduction, and of course, the immune system. This is where they play an important role in combating allergies, showing good results in fighting other diseases such as asthma and rhinitis.

Our body acquires these minerals from the foods we eat. However, our diet should be well balanced in order to receive the right nutrients. To fight allergies, your body requires higher amounts, and it is recommended to take nutritional supplements containing these elements.

Therapists prescribe appropriate and personalized treatment for each patient. The most essential minerals for treating allergic rhinitis are copper, potassium, manganese, sulfur, and silicon.

- **Bach Flowers**

The emotional state of a person can trigger an allergic crisis. The presence of allergens is not necessary to provoke an attack of sneezing, which can be triggered by depression or stress. As in the case of asthma sufferers, when you have rhinitis, you need to try to lead a stress-free life.

Bach Flowers can greatly help reduce stress, and the World Health Organization recognized their effectiveness in 1976.

A few drops of these flower essences help regulate our energy levels and overcome negative emotions. The supervision of a therapist is necessary to help you find solutions. There are thirty-two remedies used in this treatment, each of which corresponds to a particular characteristic or emotional state. Walnut, for example, can help with rhinitis by improving and protecting our immune system.

The role of the therapist, who will help you find solutions, is essential.

- **Reflexology**

Like the organs in the body, the nose and sinuses also have reflex points on the foot. A gentle foot massage is not only pleasant, but also has many therapeutic benefits including decongestion.

The points for the chest, lungs, and bronchi are located just below the five fingers at the top of the palms, and the point for the nose is located on the big toes.

The reflexologist will stress those areas, but also work the rest of the foot, especially focusing on the points connected to the liver and intestine.

You can gently massage your fingers daily, and massaging your hands and feet will help you relax and improve your energy flow, helping you to feel much better all around. When massaging your hand, the fingers should all be massaged upward except for the thumb, which should be massaged downward. This simple operation can be performed any time, anywhere. Although feet contain many sensitive pressure points, hands are more convenient to massage whenever you want.

- **Yoga**

There is a technique called Jala Neti Yoga, which is very effective for those who suffer from rhinitis. This Hindu name is for a simple nasal wash, but its particular method provides excellent results, as it not only cleans but also stimulates the nasal sinuses and the body in general.

Dietetics centers and yoga schools sell "neti pots," which is the vessel used to administer the saltwater solution to the nose. The experts can tell you the correct amount of water and unrefined sea salt that you should use to perform the irrigations. The water goes in one nostril and out the other, as if it were a siphon. It has been found that continuous use is highly effective in the treatment of rhinitis.

Furthermore, the practice of yoga is also very beneficial, as it allows you to balance the body physically and spiritually. The relaxation and breathing techniques help raise awareness of our bodies and our minds and strengthen us at all levels.

Allergic Dermatitis

Allergic dermatitis, also known as "eczema" or "atopic dermatitis," is a skin disease that affects a large number of people.

Atopic dermatitis is common in small children. Children tend to overcome their symptoms over about three years, but if it persists into adulthood, it is difficult to find a solution.

Dermatitis often accompanies asthma, hay fever, and other allergic diseases, and visibly worsens when the patient goes through a time of emotional stress. The person suffering from dermatitis is usually very sensitive and the body expresses stress and negative emotions through the skin.

The skin is the largest organ of our body and is not only subjected to external factors, such as allergens or environmental pollution, but also is particularly influenced by everything that happens in our mind and body.

What causes allergic dermatitis? As in the case of asthma and allergic rhinitis, conventional medicine ignores the root cause of this disorder on skin and the condition can become chronic.

Atopic dermatitis is an extreme skin sensitivity that people who have a history of allergies in your own person or family tend to develop.

Many babies suffer from atopic dermatitis, especially in the face and the area in contact with the diaper. They often overcome it by adolescence. However, there are children who suffer from these ailments into adulthood. Allergy tests can confirm the diagnosis of eczema in most cases, although there are types of dermatitis that share symptoms with eczema but are not allergic reactions.

Is atopic dermatitis an allergy?

Conventional medicine proved years ago that atopic eczema was not really an allergy, but rather a hypersensitivity, because there was no relationship between IgE antibodies and dermatitis, and there were no mast cells (cells related to IgE) found in the skin.

➤

The scientific community found that the allergens that usually cause asthma, rhinitis, or digestive problems also have the ability to trigger an eczema outbreak. This was until 1986, when the Dutch scientist Carla Bruynzeel-Koomen discovered the cause of atopic eczema. They are Langerhans cells, which devour foreign substances found in the skin.

The study showed that the skin of patients with atopic dermatitis has a disproportionate number of Langerhans cells that are loaded with IgE antibodies. These cells "capture" the allergenic proteins and other immunological cells that trigger the dermatitis.

This discovery earned Bruynzeel-Koomen an award from the European Academy of Allergy and Clinical Immunology in 1987.

There is also contact dermatitis, where the allergic reaction is much more limited and is caused by contact with the allergen. The most common allergens are usually certain metals, latex, synthetic garments, chemical products such as formaldehyde, wood, chlorine, or detergents.

If you have very dry skin and suffer from any allergies, or if a family member has it, you're very likely to suffer outbreaks of dermatitis or eczema throughout your life.

Even if you have a predisposition to allergies, your skin will stay healthy if you keep away from the allergen that causes you to have a reaction. However, it is not always possible, as in the case of mites or pollen, and we also do not always know which substance will cause the reaction.

How does it manifest? In atopic dermatitis or allergic skin, a response is often pervasive. The skin becomes dry, and dander is caused by the inflammatory process. The most obvious symptoms are redness, itching, formation of vesicles, and exudation of them. The affected area becomes itchy and inflamed, causing the patient to scratch the area which, in turn, makes the skin become swollen and leathery.

Continuously scratching the inflamed area can also provoke an infection and make the symptoms more complicated. These areas are often on the face, ankles, knees, and elbows, but can appear anywhere in the body.

Although eczema is considered a benign disorder, sufferers often have sleeping problems due to intense itching. This strains the body and causes nervousness, irritability, and fatigue.

Treatment. First, given that there is a higher rate of dermatitis in small children, we should address any relation to breastfeeding. Of course, the best thing you can feed a baby is breast milk. It is an excellent preventive treatment for allergies in newborns. It has been shown that children who breastfeed tend not to suffer atopic dermatitis. In addition, among mothers who do not drink cow's milk, the percentage of children free from eczema is much higher.

Breastfeeding is essential for strengthening the immune system of the child and it is advisable to nurse the child as long as possible. Within the body of the mother lays the secret of good health, and breastfeeding is a responsibility that all mothers should assume, unless there is some medical impairment that does not allow for it.

As far as the treatment of the disease is concerned, in atopic and contact eczema it is critical, as in all diseases of allergic origin, to try to avoid any contact with the allergen and maintain a positive mental and emotional attitude. Stress and negative emotions are almost as harmful as the most potent allergen.

Also, you should follow some basic rules to eliminate any agent that can irritate your skin. You must take them into account in the case of contact eczema in areas of your skin that touch clothing.

It is best not to use wool or synthetic materials, because people with dermatitis do not usually tolerate these well. You should instead wear silk or cotton clothing. Sometimes clothes are 100 percent cotton but the seams have been sewn with synthetic thread and can cause allergies. You can identify them because they look clearer. In addition, you should wash clothing several times before wearing them to remove the chemicals that are used in the factory, and it is very important that you do it at home because the dry cleaner also uses chemicals that tend to produce irritation. You should use neutral soap or soap flakes because regular detergents, including biological ones, often cause reactions. If you are allergic to cotton clothes too, this could be due to textile dyes.

Shoes can also produce skin reactions in people. The leather undergoes several processes with chemicals. In addition, the other footwear materials use formaldehyde, which can easily provoke contact eczema in people who are sensitive to the chemicals. The solution is to wear thick socks to insulate your feet from the leather or plastic.

It is also important that you use cotton bedding rather than wool blankets or quilts. The best choices are a mattress or futon made from plant material and a cotton blanket.

Tap water can produce itching due to chlorine and other additives. As it is difficult to wash with spring water in the urban environment and using bottled water can be expensive, it is best to take showers that are as short as possible and only on alternate days. Avoid all cosmetics except those that are completely free of perfumes and chemical additives. Consult your dietary center on products according to your situation.

One of the most common causes of contact dermatitis is latex. You must be especially careful if you have children, because the pacifier or nipple of the bottle may cause a breakout on their face. The same can happen with teethers or toys.

Another common cause of atopic dermatitis is the chemicals that are used for making furniture, such as formaldehyde. If you have neutralized possible allergens but continue to show symptoms, it could be perhaps due to these products.

CONVENTIONAL MEDICINE

Conventional medicine treats the symptoms of the disease, rather than the origin. Doctors will often prescribe hydrocortisone creams to relieve skin inflammation, antihistamines to relieve itching, and antibiotics in cases like eczema that has been complicated by infection due to scratching.

Apart from the drawbacks of the side effects from these drugs, treatment with corticosteroids and antibiotics may alleviate symptoms, but the relief will only be temporary.

Doctors may also prescribe sleep aids, as certain symptoms may cause insomnia.

NATURAL THERAPIES

Doctors typically reserve drugs for severe cases, advising patients to use home treatments to relieve itching. They usually recommend natural or oat-based soaps, or soap substitutes, or a warm bath with two heaping tablespoons of oatmeal added to it can help soothe the skin. Take short showers, and pat the skin dry gently with a towel. Apply a natural, hypoallergenic moisturizer such as calendula ointment or vitamin E, while the skin is still damp.

If you still feel very itchy, apply ice or onion juice to the affected area.

- **Natural Diet**

  In some cases, atopic eczema is triggered by allergens such as dust mites or pollen, but statistics show there are many cases of dermatitis caused by food allergies. In the case of a food allergy, it is most effective to avoid the food triggering the reaction, and to follow a healthy and balanced diet.

  However, there are other cases of atopic dermatitis that have no clear origin and that many therapists say often cover up a food intolerance. Nutritionists recommend an elimination diet.

  This type of diet should not be used along with any other treatment for skin conditions, not even a natural therapy.

The aim is to observe the symptoms that manifest them-selves. If you are suffering from a food intolerance, your skin will heal and stop itching. These results can be quite dramatic in children.

The first step in an elimination diet requires about five days of completely avoiding the foods suspected of causing the reaction. Limit your diet to a few foods that certainly do not cause allergies, such as rice, for example. To effec-tively pursue this treatment, it is essential to count on the advice of a nutritionist.

After spending five days on a basal diet, patients often see a remarkable improvement in the condition of their skin. Next, they should begin to reintroduce the foods they had elimi-nated, watching for any reaction in their skin. If one of the foods causes an intolerance, the eczema will flare up again. It may happen after a few minutes, or after a day or two. These results will help the nutritionist design a healthy diet plan for you that will keep your skin clear of inflammation and itching. Some indications that your skin is healing include changes in coloration (the skin going from a deep red to a bluish red) and a change in texture caused by the shedding of the old skin to make way for the new, healthy skin.

You can also help identify a food intolerance by taking the tests mentioned in previous chapters. Being tested for the 120 most common food allergies can help narrow down your list of "forbidden foods" and find solutions to your atopic problems. Another factor to keep in mind when fol-lowing a balanced diet is your vitamin intake. Make sure to consume fruits and leafy greens, brewer's yeast, and whole grains, all of which contain high levels of vitamins B and C and calcium. Vitamin B is also found in eggs and milk, but we recommend that you avoid these products because they are also highly allergenic.

Marine and freshwater algae are great natural sources of vitamins, minerals, and trace elements. These aquatic plants provide us with a wealth of very important minerals in a much higher concentration than other natural foods. They are an important part of your diet, but should be introduced in moderation because of their strong, unique flavor. They also help the body eliminate metals and toxins from its system, and keep your skin in good condition.

- **Heliotherapy**
Sunlight is the source of life, helping to synthesize vitamins and activating and strengthening the skin—in moderation, of course. If you live in a sunny climate, you can benefit greatly from a walk in the sun each day. In summer, it is best to take a walk around ten in the morning, rather than early afternoon when the sun's rays are too strong. In winter the procedure is reversed and there is nothing better than a walk in the midday sun. You must gradually increase exposure ten minutes at a time, building up to an hour over the course of a few weeks.

If your lifestyle and the climate of your region do not allow you to sunbathe, you can always use sun lamps, which provide artificial sun that has similar benefits to those of natural sunlight. However, do not give up the former if you can.

If you decide to pursue a sun treatment, it is best to choose a location near the beach. Sun in the high mountains is also very beneficial for conditions such as respiratory diseases. In addition, sunlight stimulates the metabolism, improves appetite, and boosts your immune system. However, environments by the sea are particularly suited for helping to fix skin problems, due to the higher moisture level, constant temperature, and the interaction of ultraviolet rays with iodine.

Obviously, if you suffer from sun allergies you should not follow any of these therapies, except very gradually and under the strict control of a specialist.

Dermatologists and therapists have noted that atopic eczema improves with exposure to sunlight and the symptoms of cutaneous dryness, scaling, and itching, are relieved. This is because the sun activates blood circulation, giving you a greater supply of oxygen and nutrients to the skin. It also stimulates melanin, which also strengthens the skin.

The sun stimulates the secretion of important hormones as it reaches the hypothalamus through our eyes. As you know, this gland is the control center for many functions of our body and mind, so sunlight also provides us important benefits.

- **Homeopathy**
  Atopic eczema can be improved significantly thanks to constitutional remedies, so it is essential you choose a good homeopath who can make an accurate diagnosis, not just to help discern the appropriate constitutional remedy, but to avoid a major "homeopathic aggravation" that could impair the health of your skin early in treatment.

- **Phytotherapy and poultices**
  Herbs can also help you to try and overcome dermatitis. Also, they not only provide benefits in the form of infusion, but they can calm your itching and reduce inflammation if you apply them topically, that is, directly on the affected area. Herbal poultices have anti-inflammatory, emollient, antibacterial, and antipruritic effects, due to their active ingredients.
  Your herbalist will know how to advise you on which different species can improve your condition and how you should prepare the herbs for treatment.

Nettles	Reduce itching.
Mullein	Prevents infection. Boil the leaves and wash the area with the infused water.

➤

Borage	Tones the skin. You can take it orally or apply an infusion topically after bathing.
Laurel	Prevents infection and regenerates the skin. Macerate in olive oil and apply to your skin, or add leaves to your bath water.
Malva	An emollient applied with a cold compress soaked in an infusion of leaves and flowers.
Elder	Has anti-inflammatory properties. Apply a poultice of young leaves to your skin.
Arnica	Has analgesic, anti-inflammatory, and antibacterial properties. You can take it in an infusion, use in baths, or apply poultices to your skin.
Guava leaves	topical application improves eczema due to antibacterial and astringent qualities.
Hops	Its soothing effects aid in sleep and prevent itching that could wake you up. Also, it is very suitable for the external treatment of eczema because of its high zinc content.
Clover	Has astringent and healing properties that help restore your skin's appearance. Apply it to your skin in a poultice.

Evening primrose oil is extracted from the primrose flower. This substance has many uses in herbal medicine, including treating atopic or contact eczema. Applying primrose oil to affected areas for three to four months can relieve the itching and dryness in your skin. Its active ingredients can be equated to the anti-inflammatory creams and ointments that use corticosteroids or immunomodulators, providing a highly effective natural solution for troublesome symptoms of dermatitis.

● **Acupuncture**

The ancient healing technique of acupuncture considers disease to come from a problem with the flow of vital energy that runs through the body, and works to rebalance and restore health to the sick.

This therapy, which helps your body on the path to self-healing, is used to treat multiple disorders and diseases. Allergic contact dermatitis and is one of them.

By stimulating the appropriate acupoints, the acupuncturist helps hydrate your skin, helps reduce inflammation and itching, and helps you feel more relaxed. Acupuncture also strengthens your immune system, which helps prevent it from responding in an exaggerated way to harmless substances.

The acupuncturist will also recommend other traditional Chinese treatments, such as diet or a particular use of certain medicinal herbs that act synergistically with acupuncture and help improve your condition.

Allergic dermatitis is considered by conventional medicine to be a chronic disease. Acupuncture will not provide immediate results, but through weekly sessions you will find as you check on your skin that your symptoms will go away naturally and permanently.

● **Oligotherapy**

People with atopic eczema or contact dermatitis often have a low level of trace elements in their bodies. Although diet can provide most of these, an extra dose can help kickstart your recovery.

Important trace elements that keep your skin healthy are zinc, magnesium, selenium, and manganese. You should always consult an experienced therapist who can advise you on proper dosage.

● **Reflexology**

Although we sometimes overlook this fact, the skin is the largest organ in our body. And as such, it can be treated with reflexology to help control eczema.

This Chinese therapy works well to activate blood circulation, strengthen the immune system, and improve the emotional state through massaging pressure points in your feet and hands. The goal of reflexology is to regulate your body and skin and allow them to begin to self-heal with their own tools. Check with your therapist about the number and duration of sessions, and feel free to give yourself foot or hand massages to help relieve your eczema.

- **Yoga**
At first glance it may seem that a therapy based on movement, relaxation, and breath control cannot really help when it comes to a skin problem. However, nothing is further from the truth.

Our body and mind form a unit and are in constant communication. Everything that happens on an emotional level will reflect physically, and eczema is one of the most representative cases. And, in fact, our negative emotions, stress, nervousness, or depression can, and indeed do, exacerbate episodes of allergic dermatitis. Therefore it is very important to learn to relax, take care of our self-esteem, nurture our positive vision of life, and work and practice loving ourselves and others.

If you practice yoga on a daily basis it can rebalance your body so that it works better. It is a comprehensive tool that boosts your immune system, frees your body, and teaches you to breathe deeply to get oxygen into every last corner of your body. It is also a philosophy of life that provides serenity and inner harmony with its teachings on meditation and relaxation. All these factors can help you recover balance between your emotions and immune system.

Food Allergies and Intolerances

Food allergy and food intolerance, or pseudoallergy, differ in the origin of the disease. In food allergies, allergens from one or more foods generate an exaggerated response in our immune system, which is mediated by IgE antibodies. The allergy occurs immediately or within a few hours, and its symptoms include inflammation and itching. The symptoms can result in a number of allergic diseases, including asthma, rhinitis, eczema, and anaphylactic shock.

However, in the case of an intolerance, no allergen triggers the immune response with IgE antibodies. This is a reaction to certain proteins found in the food, due to hypersensitivity in the metabolism. There are certain foods that, more or less rapidly, generate inflammation and pruritus—symptoms identical to those brought on by an allergy. This explains why you can have asthma, rhinitis, or eczema without positive results from allergy testing.

In the first chapter, we described in detail the mechanisms of both allergies and intolerances. In addition, we've provided an overview of the most common foods that can cause these ailments, focusing on lactose and gluten. Food allergies and intolerances can cause uncomfortable symptoms such as inflammation of the digestive track. We will provide information about both natural and conventional treatments to help relieve symptoms and prevent future reactions.

How allergies and food intolerances manifest themselves. As we have explained, allergies and food intolerances can cause any of the diseases we have described in the previous pages: asthma, rhinitis, and dermatitis. However, only food allergies can cause serious problems or anaphylactic shock, especially if they are caused by nuts, eggs, fish, and shellfish. Reactions do not always occur immediately; sometimes they occur hours after eating even just a small amount of the food in question.

Besides respiratory allergies or skin problems, they can also cause other digestive symptoms such as diarrhea, abdominal pain, or intestinal gas. Still other complaints related to intestinal problems and whose origin may be due to an allergy or food intolerance include fatigue, migraines, dry mouth, canker sores, obesity, chills, psoriasis, itchy irritated eyes or mouth, muscle aches, backaches, depression, anxiety, hyperactivity, inability to concentrate, fluid retention, palpitations, joint pain, and many more.

Symptoms can be reduced if the foods that produce reactions are removed from your diet, but it is always necessary to properly restore the intestinal flora, as it has suffered considerable damage from the reactions. The difficult part is finding the food causing the problems, and any foods that could be causing a cross-reaction. For example, if you have an intolerance to onions, it is not enough to remove onions from your diet. Garlic belongs to the same family and may sooner or later end up causing the same symptoms.

We have mentioned before the importance of keeping the intestine in an optimal state. Intestinal flora problems leave the door open to allergies and food intolerances because they cause leaky gut syndrome, which allows whole proteins to pass into the bloodstream and cause reactions. It is essential that your diet and lifestyle promote good intestinal flora that will help prevent metabolization problems and diseases.

It is also important to keep stress under control. If you are suffering anxiety, your digestive system cannot properly perform its function. Poorly digested food irritates the lining of the intestine, causing it to become permeable. Even if your diet is healthy, your intestinal flora will cause you the same problems when you eat problematic foods. The substances that your gut cannot digest well will enter the bloodstream, causing problems in the liver, kidneys, and of course, the immune system. It is therefore essential to try to change your lifestyle and daily habits to reduce stress. Many therapies can help with this, from reiki to yoga, through meditation or tai-chi. You can practice these methods in the comfort of your own home, making them a part of your daily schedule to help treat your body well and develop emotional stability.

Lactose intolerance. Cow's milk and all its derivatives are recognized producers of mucous, and therefore are not suitable for people with allergy problems.

Cow's milk contains two substances — casein and lactose — that can cause allergic reactions or types of food intolerance. Lactose intolerance is one of the most common food pseudoallergies.

As we have explained previously, milk contains a sugar called "lactose," which in many cases produces a condition known as "lactose intolerance." While this sugar is not detrimental to our bodies, our digestive system requires the presence of the enzyme lactase, which turns the lactose into galactose and glucose. The problem is that this enzyme, which is produced in the intestinal mucosa, begins decreasing in levels from birth, and there are children who are born with a deficiency in this enzyme. There are also diseases that affect lactase molecules and deplete them, causing gastrointestinal diseases such as celiac.

This is one reason why our bodies sometimes do not absorb cow's milk and we become likely to develop a food intolerance. It is sometimes apparent in newborns, but other times, it doesn't develop until adulthood.

Yogurt does not cause lactose intolerance because yogurts contain very little lactose, and the bacteria that turn milk into yogurt possess the necessary enzymes to digest lactose. The digestive process begins in the yogurt itself and helps the intestine absorb nutrients more easily. Its viscous texture also facilitates digestion by slowing gastric emptying. However, it must be naturally made yogurt, without chemical additives or industrial processes. We recommend that you make your own yogurt at home to ensure that the bacteria fermenting the yogurt are alive.

Lactose intolerance prevents milk products from being digested, causing them to remain in the large intestine where they ferment. This process produces lactic acid, short-chain fatty acids, hydrogen, carbon dioxide, and methane. Their presence in our body causes diarrhea, flatulence, abdominal pain, abdominal distension, weight loss, malnutrition, allergies, and problems in the skin, digestive track, immune system, and so on.

There are three diagnostic methods to detect the presence of lactose intolerance. One test has the patient drink milk and take blood samples every half hour to see if there has been an increase in blood glucose from the digestion of lactose. Another test examines the levels of hydrogen in the breath after ingesting lactose. A third form of diagnosis tests the acid in feces. A biopsy of the small intestine can also check the levels of lactase in the intestinal mucosa, but is used as a last resort because it is an invasive procedure.

The most effective treatment of lactose intolerance is to entirely eliminate products containing lactose from your diet. There are many other substitutes to help supplement your diet if you have removed dairy from your diet. Milk provides us with calcium, but there are many other healthy sources of calcium that you can consume instead. Tofu, soy milk fortified with calcium, soy yogurt, leafy greens, parsley, watercress, chard, broccoli, turnips, almonds, sesame seeds, tahini (sesame paste), and tempeh (made from fermented soybeans), all contain high levels of calcium. Sunbathing can help supply your body with vitamin D, which helps your metabolism bind calcium to the bone.

Eliminating Lactose.

It is not always easy to remove dairy derivatives from your diet, because the food industry uses them in many ways and in a huge number of products. This means you have to read all food labels and discard any that mention any of the following components:

- Instant Milk, nonfat dry.
- Margarine.
- Milk derivatives.
- Butter.
- Casein hydrolyzate.

➤

- Serum.
- Cream.
- Curd.
- Cheese.

Other food products that may incorporate lactose among its components are:

- Soups or purees enriched with milk or milk derivatives.
- Fresh and fermented cheese.
- Deli meat containing dairy products.
- Pastry and fried meat, fish or poultry containing dairy products.
- Eggs prepared with milk or milk derivatives.
- Egg substitutes, for example, those involved in smoothies, puddings
- Food made from milk or milk products, such as mashed potatoes, prepared pasta dishes, etc.
- Creams and purees made with milk or milk products, such as creamed spinach.
- Bakery products containing milk or milk derivatives: pancakes, muffins, cakes, cookies, pastries, toast, etc.
- Precooked or ready-to-eat foods containing milk derivatives.
- Protein-enriched cereal.
- Butter, margarine, and cream dairy products.
- Salad dressings and mayonnaise with milk or milk derivatives.
- Milk-based drinks, such as smoothies.
- Milk chocolate, cream, or cream sauce and gratin dishes.
- Fried or battered foods.
- Chocolate-coated tablets.

Also, you should know that certain drugs are made with lactose, so they can cause symptoms. You should always read labels carefully.

After eliminating lactose from your diet, you must very slowly reincorporate fiber and fats, because they are difficult to digest.

You should drink plenty of fluids, and eat light meals to avoid overloading your digestive system. In addition, we recommend that you consume plenty of prebiotics and probiotics to help restore your intestinal flora.

Prebiotics and Probiotics

You have probably heard of prebiotics and probiotics if you have an interest in natural nutrition and healthy living habits.

Lactose intolerance is one of the many problems that can seriously affect your intestinal flora, and probiotics and prebiotics are substances that can provide a significant boost in your recovery. Probiotics nourish the intestinal flora, and pre-biotics help reset it. Prebiotics are found in plant foods such as wheat, asparagus, garlic, leeks, onions, beets, chicory root, and artichokes. The most common are called inulin and fructooligosaccharides. Foods with a high content of prebiotics are resistant to digestion, causing them to ferment in the large intestine and produce short-chain fatty acids that nourish the colonocytes (cells of the large intestine). Sometimes this fermentation causes flatulence, so it could be best to wait until you feel healthy to begin incorporating prebiotics into your diet.

Probiotic foods (or promoters of life) contain beneficial bacteria, especially lactobacilli and bifidobacteria. They can be consumed as a nutritional supplement or in yogurt. These bacteria are very beneficial to people who suffer from lactose intolerance because if their intestinal flora is in good condition, in the mucosal inflammation is reduced and symptoms can be relieved.

By combining prebiotic and probiotic foods, you can reduce bowel hypersensitivity and replenish and maintain gut flora. You will raise your levels of beneficial bacteria.

Natural therapies can help alleviate the symptoms caused by this intolerance. The options are varied and you can combine more than one for a speedy recovery.

Herbal teas can help you control the inflammation. Neuropathy can help find the right diet and oligotherapy is very useful for recovering your nutritional balance. In many other conditions, homeopathy, acupuncture, reflexology, and other energetic therapies will help to restore the pH balance of your body. Disciplines such as yoga, psychotherapy, relaxation, or breathing exercises will teach you how to reduce stress, a factor of great importance in lactose intolerance.

Gluten intolerance. This foodborne ailment, also known as "celiac disease" or "gluten-induced enteropathy," is a major intestinal disorder. Its origin is an intolerance to a protein—gluten—found in a large number of grains such as wheat, rye, barley, and oats.

It is a relatively new disease, present in areas of the world where the diet contains a significant presence of cereals.

The effects of gluten intolerance manifest themselves in a number of symptoms that are caused by an alteration of the villi of the intestinal mucosa. Our body is nourished by the food we eat, which is digested by the small intestine. The villi that make up this system create a larger surface in the digestive track, increasing its capacity for absorption. Gluten damages these villi, and in severe cases, can shrink what should be long stems into small bumps. This reduction in absorption capacity can cause disorders such as diarrhea, fatigue, abdominal pain, irritability, malnutrition, and weight loss.

Gluten intolerance occurs in both adults and children, and in the case of children, can cause growth problems due to malnutrition. It can produce dehydration, bruises in the skin, gastrointestinal bleeding, and fluid retention in the form of edema.

However, this disease does not always show these symptoms. As there is a hereditary component, the doctor may often test the whole family to see if the patient is the only one affected, and many cases of celiac people can be in an early stage of the disease without knowing. Many people suffer from celiac

165

disease without realizing it. Among other symptoms that can be caused by gluten intolerance are: constipation, short stature, rickets, osteoporosis, spontaneous fractures, bone pain, alteration in the enamel of the teeth, recurring canker sores, dermatitis herpetiformis, migraines, hair loss, neuralgia, depression, epilepsy, anemia, bleeding, miscarriage, infertility, arthritis, and joint pain.

It is a condition that can occur at any age and has serious consequences if left untreated. As of now, it is incurable, and the only truly effective remedy is to completely remove all traces of foods that cause symptoms. Following a gluten-free diet can quickly regenerate the intestinal mucosa and restore the villi to their normal size.

The only definitive diagnosis is provided by a series of biopsies, but you can easily tell if you suffer from a gluten intolerance if your symptoms notably improve after eliminating problem foods from your diet.

However, although the remedy might seem simple, the fact is that maintaining a gluten-free diet is often an arduous task, as in Western society, gluten is found in a vast number of food products.

For a celiac it is essential to know which foods contain gluten, as it is not always clearly indicated on food labels. The food industry is increasing its range of gluten-free foods, such as specialty breads, pastries, and pastas, as an alternative to their natural forms. The drawback is that, although the appearance and taste of these foods is fairly accurate, they are often quite expensive. There are many associations that support celiac patients, both with psychological support for patients and their families, and with advice on which food products are recommended and which are not. They have drawn up lists of gluten-free foods that are sold in dietetic centers.

Below, we provide a list of foods that are prohibited, tolerated, and allowed so you can navigate food products, preferably along with the advice of a specialist.

PROHIBITED FOODS

- Bread and wheat, rye, barley, and oat flour
- Wheatmeal
- Pasta, baked goods, cookies, and pastries
- Processed foods that contain any flour
- Prepared or canned food whose label does not specify that it does not contain gluten
- Chocolate (unless it is gluten-free)
- Beverages made with milk and cereals: malt, beer, water, barley, and oat milk

PERMISSIBLE FOODS ONLY IF THE LABEL STATES THAT IT DOES NOT CONTAIN GLUTEN

- Deli meat
- Processed cheese
- Paté
- Canned foods
- Candy
- Nougat
- Marzipan
- Instant coffee
- Tea

GLUTEN-FREE FOODS

- Milk
- Other dairy products (cheese, butter, cottage cheese, cream)
- Meat
- Fish
- Seafood
- Eggs
- Fruit
- Vegetables
- Legumes
- Rice
- Corn
- Tapioca (flour and starch)

NATURAL TREATMENT OF ALLERGIES

- Sugar
- Honey
- Oil
- Margarine
- Salt
- Vinegar
- Pepper
- Yeast
- Food coloring
- Coffee, whole beans or ground
- Herbal teas
- Carbonated soft drinks

Note: These foods are allowed in their natural state, as long as you do not buy canned foods.

Treatment of allergies and food intolerances. As with all allergies and intolerances, the best treatment is to remove the allergen that causes the reaction from your life. In the case of food allergens, you can exercise more effective control over them than over pollen or mites, for example.

However, the problem is often in knowing which foods are causing your symptoms. Allergy testing and food intolerance tests can help greatly with this, although it may also be useful to ask for the help of a nutritionist to find which food is responsible for your illness.

If you obtain an accurate diagnosis, another obstacle to overcome is that of cross-reactions. It is very important that you know all the foods that are associated with giving you allergic reactions. Although in this book we have described some of the major food allergens, you should seek expert advice to gain even more information about this problem.

As with other allergic conditions, there are several ways to tackle your illness. In all cases, you must first try to find out which allergen triggers your reactions, and then choose your preferred method of treatment. Conventional medicine gives you relief from the symptoms with drugs; these drugs come with side effects. Natural therapies are very different because they help you rebalance your body and boost your immune system, while seeking a solution to troublesome symptoms.

You and only you can make decisions about your health. But whatever path you choose, it is imperative that you follow the treatment to the letter, with responsibility and conviction.

Finally, reducing stress and maintaining a positive attitude are key factors in your recovery and can help you to feel better emotionally and achieve the inner peace and harmony that your body needs to recover.

CONVENTIONAL MEDICINE

As for conventional medicine, drugs that can help improve your symptoms are antihistamines and anti-inflammatory medicines. The combination depends on the repercussions that allergies may have on your body and varies depending on whether it is asthma, rhinitis, or dermatitis.

If the problem is isolated, in your gut for example, it is highly recommended that you follow a specific diet designed by an allergist to maintain your digestive system and to offset symptoms by eliminating the food or foods that cause these symptoms.

There is no immunotherapy, or allergy shots, designed for food allergy.

NATURAL THERAPIES

This approach to health is a holistic approach, that is, geared toward both your physical and emotional welfare. Your ultimate goal is self-healing your body and this approach will provide your body with the necessary tools to achieve this.

It is usually a slower process but with surprising results in many cases. Its goal is to get to the root of the problem—an arduous task due to the imbalance in the immune system caused by allergic reactions, one of the most important systems in our body. There are many cases of patients who choose natural therapies to heal after trying conventional medication. They usually suffer from chronic allergies and it is impossible to find quick solutions to these ailments. Natural therapies not only help patients to feel better, but they also help you to regain balance in your body.

It is likely that your therapist will recommend combining therapies or seeing several different specialists. The secret lies in the synergy between different natural treatments. Combining methods increases their collective power and shortens the path to your recovery.

- **Natural Diet**

There is no doubt that a healthy diet is the foundation of a healthy body. A diet full of fruits and vegetables helps your body absorb necessary nutrients.

However, in the case of food allergies that affect the digestive system, your diet becomes an even more important factor, because your guts are in poor condition. Because of this, we should not consume products that damage your intestinal flora, such as milk and dairy products, sugar, coffee, or alcoholic beverages.

You should also remove foods that are high in histamine from your diet, or consume them only in moderation. This is especially important when you are not feeling well because they can enhance your IgE response. These foods include chocolate, tomatoes, fish, nuts, cheese, pineapple, strawberries, and eggs.

Also avoid processed foods, as they often contain a cocktail of chemical additives that do not benefit you at all. You should eat light, whole foods of good quality. Talk to your nutritionist, and treat your diet as though it were a medicinal regimen, as diet is very important to help restore your health.

In addition, it is essential not to smoke because nicotine contains chemical components that irritate the mucosa and prevent proper absorption of the nutrients that your body needs.

If your allergy prevents you from eating certain foods, naturopaths can recommend others that replace the nutritional deficit. You can even take nutritional supplements to help balance your diet. They work very well and are very useful in preventing deficiencies in nutrients.

Once your symptoms are under control, your body needs to receive necessary nutrients through your diet, since it is the most natural and healthiest way to feel good.

Phytotherapy

The role of this therapy when treating a food allergy is similar to that of conventional medicine, as it is based on certain medicinal plants with anti-inflammatory and anti-histaminic properties.

Therefore, you can benefit from symptomatic relief without resorting to drugs.

Although we provide a list of the main options, it is always advisable to turn to your herbalist so you can prepare a mixture that fits your condition and your lifestyle. You will soon be enjoying a quiet moment in front of a steaming cup of herbal tea.

Green anise	inhibits intestinal fermentation and combats flatulence and spasms.
Comfrey	has antihistaminic properties. Usually prepared in decoction.
Ginko biloba	a recognized anti-inflammatory whose stimulating properties make it a digestive tonic.

> | | |
> |---|---|
> | Chamomile | has soothing and antispasmodic properties, which is very helpful in cases of irritable bowel syndrome. |
> | Melisa | a powerful antispasmodic. |
> | Mint | has analgesic properties and helps in digestion |

- **Oligotherapy**

As mentioned above, our body cannot produce certain minerals that it needs to stay in perfect balance. These substances are involved in many of our bodily functions, but especially to help regulate and balance our body. They are also of vital importance to the intestine, and oligotherapists can prescribe you essential minerals to help you prevent allergic reactions. The most important are iron, copper, iodine, manganese, selenium, zinc, chromium, cobalt, fluorine, lithium, nickel, and silicon, but it is essential that the specialist assesses your status and customizes the treatment. Good professional advice and oligotherapy will help your recovery.

- **Homeopathy**

In the case of allergies, whatever their manifestation, homeopathy provides solutions to get your body back into balance and to begin the process of self-healing.

Homeopaths can prescribe a constitutional remedy—a treatment that has no side effects, although there may be a "homeopathic aggravation" early in the treatment.

This symptom indicates that the remedy is beginning to rebalance your body and this reaction shows that the remedy is appropriate.

Furthermore, there are specific remedies that the homeopath can prescribe to relieve the symptoms of inflammatory bowel disease.

● **Acupuncture**

This ancient practice is very useful in treating inflammation in your gut and improving your digestion. With the help of an experienced acupuncturist, the patient can repair their digestive system and feel better.

In addition, acupuncture helps you rebalance the whole body, so it is not just a therapy to solve your most obvious symptoms, but also to achieve overall recovery of your immune system.

Relax and follow the advice of the specialist. They can recommend a diet tailored to your symptoms, and some herbs to further improve your health. These are the three basic pillars of traditional Chinese medicine, and their synergy has provided solutions for people for the last three thousand years.

● **Yoga**

As food allergies cause digestive problems, you may feel a general malaise. There are various yoga asanas that stimulate the digestive system and help aid in digestion.

Yoga also provides harmony and inner peace through breathing exercises and relaxation postures. The former are very important because they help oxygenate your body, and the latter also are essential in the treatment of food allergies because stress and nerves have a direct effect on the digestive system. It is essential that you control your stress and try to lead a quiet, orderly life. Rest and a positive attitude are also crucial ingredients in your improvement, and this therapy can help significantly.

We are confident that you're going to start therapy and create a lifestyle that provides you with physical and psychological benefits, and a comfortable environment.